EPI-PALEO RX

The Prescription for Disease Reversal and Optimal Health

By Dr. Jack Kruse

Epi-paleo Rx

ISBN 978-0-9890577-3-8

Library of Congress Control Number: 2013934829

Published by:

Optimized Life PLC
Dr. Jack Kruse
kruseschedule@gmail.com
jackkruse.com

Cover photography and book design by fawcettphotodesign.com

Contents

About The Author

DR. JACK KRUSE

Dr. Jack Kruse is a respected neurosurgeon and CEO of Optimized Life, a health and wellness company dedicated to helping patients avoid the healthcare burdens we typically encounter as we age. He is a member of the American Association of Neurological Surgeons, the Congress of Neurologic Surgeons, and Age Management Medicine Group.

As a neurosurgeon, Dr. Kruse's research has been published in respected dental and medical journals. His popular blog, www.JackKruse.com, gets over 150,000 unique worldwide visitors per month from countries like Australia, Germany, Russia, and Zambia (Africa).

Introduction

Until the late 1800s, the leading causes of death were infectious diseases-tuberculosis, pneumonia and syphilis. We can credit antibiotics and other developments for limiting their risk of death.

However, chronic Neolithic diseases such as cancer, Alzheimer's disease, heart disease and others are now the leading causes of death, despite improvements in sanitation and personal hygiene. While we successfully battled infectious diseases, we allowed industrialized food and corporations to marginalize small farmer and lower the quality and nutrient density of food.

These food conglomerates favor industrial seed oils due to their lower costs. As heart attacks became the number-one cause of death in the 40s and 50s, the lipid hypothesis, which links heart disease to saturated fat, took root and campaigns promoting these profitable seed oils began.

The lipid hypothesis became medical dogma, cemented it in the national consciousness by the USDA Food Pyramid and media attention. This is well chronicled in many books, including Good Calories, Bad Calories by Gary Taubes, Michael Pollan's In Defense of Food, and Anthony Colpo's book The Great Cholesterol Con, a book that challenges everything you think you know about heart disease.

During my first class in medical school, one of my biochemistry professors told us he was required to teach the lipid hypothesis even though he believed the data was badly flawed. In those days we received less than 10 hours of nutrition lectures in medical school. This was chronicled in 1985 in a landmark paper called Nutrition Education in U.S. Medical Schools by the National Research Council. Because of that paper and my teacher's warning, I read about nutrition on my own. I went to the biochemistry department to speak with several doctoral students about and they gave me a book called Pure, White and Deadly by John Yudkin, MD. I remember reading it and realizing I was eating everything Yudkin said not to. The book was radical compared to how I was brought up to think about foods. Unfortunately, I forgot about my teacher's talk during my remaining years in medical school. The first two years of learning about the human body in medical school are like drinking water from an open fire hydrant. Even an optimal brain will forget details due to the shear volume of data, yet these first two years are when physicians learn 95 percent of the basic science that underpins the practice and art of medicine. My teacher's comments registered but were not clinically significant at the time-I was only concerned about excelling on the exam.

After my internship year in general surgery, I began to see the wisdom in my teacher's words. The dogma surrounding medicine is hard to fathom until you have lived through it first hand. I am at a loss as to why more physicians do not question many of the beliefs shoved down our throats when the treatments are clearly ineffective.

However, I kept these concerns to myself because I didn't want to rock the boat as a resident and was in no position to change anything. Instead, I was hoping to complete a mentally, physically, and emotionally brutal neurosurgery postdoctoral program. At that time, survival meant more than finding ultimate truths.

During my fifth year of residency I caught a breather during a short stint of clinical research and realized how the system enforces dogma. I listened to a talk by a seasoned vascular surgeon about the causes of atherosclerosis. In the first part of his lecture, he implicated saturated fats and oxidized cholesterol as the culprits of the disease. But during the latter half, he said as he had gotten older he realized the disease he made a career of could not be cured by surgery. In fact, he said it could not be cured by medicine at all because of money, politics, and the industrial food complex, and because medicine had become lazy about distinguishing between causation and correlation in published research. His final slide pointed the gun directly at a declining diet in the United States over the last 100 years as a cause for heart disease.

This talk watered the seed my earlier teacher had first planted. I spoke to this vascular surgeon at length during the last 18 months of my neurosurgical training. Shortly thereafter, an article appeared in the Atlantic called "Lies, Damned Lies, and Medical Science." In this article, Professor John Ioannidis, MD, PhD questioned whether drug companies manipulated published research to make their drugs look good. These drugs and treatments form the backbone of allopathic medicine. This article forced me to question much of what I had been taught about medicine, and how business, money, and politics affected medical decisions.

I then searched for evidence to support my intuition. I looked at the top 10 causes of death and the top market caps of medical stocks. The results were startling. It appeared the explosive growth of Neolithic diseases that killed millions of Americans and Europeans were linked to who profited from them. These were the statistics I found then:

The Top Ten Causes of Death In The United States of America

1. Heart disease: 652,486
2. Cancer: 553,888
3. Stroke: 150,074
4. Respiratory Disorders: 121,987
5. All Accidents: 112,012
6. Diabetes: 73,138
7. Alzheimer's: 69,965
8. Influenza and pneumonia: 59,664
9. Kidney failure: 42,480
10. Blood poisoning: 33,373

Then I reviewed the market capitalization of stocks for the business that provided bullets for the war on these diseases. Generally, those who fare best in wars are those who stay neutral and sell their products to both sides. I found the revenues of giant multinational corporations that produce a large chunk of the world's pharmaceuticals, chemicals, and agrochemicals rose exponentially along with Neolithic diseases.

1. Cardinal Health (healthcare): $47.9 billion
2. Merck (pharmaceuticals): $47.7 billion
3. Pfizer (pharmaceuticals): $32.3 billion
4. Glaxo Smith Kline (pharmaceuticals): $29.5 billion

5. Bayer (pharmaceuticals): $27.1 billion
6. United Health Group (healthcare): $23.4 billion
7. Bristol-Myers Squibb (pharmaceuticals): $21.7 billion
8. Pharmacia (pharmaceuticals): $19.3 billion
9. Novartis (pharmaceuticals): $18.9 billion
10. Amerisource Bergen (healthcare): $15.8 billion
11. WellPoint Health Networks (healthcare): $12.4 billion

(Source: Forbes 500, "2002 Revenue")

For me, the coincidence was a bit too convenient. So I decided to take my suspicions further and look at the market caps of stocks in the industrial farm complex. I got through two prospectuses from Monsanto and Potash when I realized I had found an inconvenient truth. It appeared to me that all Neolithic diseases are tied to the people who make our food and then treat us for the diseases they cause. This rise in chronic disease has also coincided with the rise in industrial farming, and I learned about the routine dosing of animals with growth hormones and antibiotics. I read several articles in the Wall Street Journal about how profitable it was for farmers to feed animals from our government-subsidized grain stockpile, and about the federal mandates to sell these products to the world. The entire picture had been painted for me as to how large volumes of people could get sick from the same diseases, and why things happened the way they did the last 100 years in our country.

What I did not have a handle on directly, however, was what in our food was the root cause of the problem. So I read more business journals about the industry. I figured if I wanted to know about these things I should focus on the money trail.

I learned about BPA, DDT, and other environmental toxins and their effects on health. I learned how we imported the idea of making sugar from corn in 1977 to replace table sugar because high-fructose corn syrup was cheaper and sweeter.

Governments around the world approved chemical weed killers, many of which have since been banned, because they were highly profitable, despite never being tested on humans. There has been no political will to regulate the genetic modification of seeds, despite the troubling animal studies and lack of human testing. The federal government is impotent because it is a partner in the same business. The federal mandate is to sell our grains to the rest of the world. The United States became the number-one producer and exporter of grains in the 20th century, and it is very profitable still today.

The simultaneous combination of all these factors made me question the integrity of the entire process from the government to the grocery stores. It seemed plausible that "safe and government-approved" chemicals and foods were the cause of many chronic diseases plaguing our country. Toxins from these foods and chemicals can stay buried in our organs and abdominal fat for years. The research is now beginning to point to these chemicals as major endocrine disruptors in humans, and abdominal fat as the source of inflammation that underpins all Neolithic diseases today.

During this time, I was sliding down my own slope of Neolithic disease by gaining weight every year as I got older. This slide accelerated after my residency when I had freedom to do whatever I wanted. The similarity in my condition and that of my patients was not lost on me, but it did little to change my habits. Truthfully, I was in denial until a physician friend of mine came to spend a week with me. He was glad to see me but his first response was that I had become a "fat ass." He then went on for an entire week how eating well was the key to staying fit and healthy. He even took me to the store and lectured me on Kerry Gold butter. It was fun, but I have to say, I thought he was California crazy! Then, four weeks later, everything changed. I tore my right knee meniscus when I stood up to give a spine talk at a meeting. This physical setback led me to learn that the torn cartilage was caused by the inflammation of my ever-growing abdominal fat. This inflammation fueled hormonal disruption and caused leptin resistance. I never learned anything about leptin in medical school. I also had no clue about how incredibly important this link would be for me personally or in my career as a surgeon. Becoming leptin resistant allowed my joints to become susceptible to a major degenerative injury, like the one I sustained from little to no activity. This injury was the catalyst to my transforming change-the picture was painted and framed in my mind that day.

I immediately went back to the library and learned all I could about the relationships between leptin, obesity, and Neolithic diseases, and I set out to learn how to re-engineer myself back to optimal. It took 18 months of constant reading of new research and data to finally understand how the food in the standard American diet was directly related to my torn meniscus, my obesity, and my declining health. It finally dawned on me that I was no different than the patients I saw in my own clinic. That spark of insight led me to transform myself, my beliefs about food and nutrition, and the way I looked at disease as a neurosurgeon, including the ones in which I specialized.

THE GENESIS OF EPI-PALEO RX

I decided to write this book after a very inspirational discussion with Primal Blueprint author Mark Sisson in December of 2011. I knew after speaking to him I needed to write about how my own transformation led me to look at disease in the clinical setting . The next morning I woke up and went through my morning ritual of waiting for the sunrise and[EF1] thinking of three new ways to improve myself. I then sat down in my robe and typed for five straight hours. I had stepped into a period of life where my thoughts were becoming actions and a dream was transforming into reality[EF2]. Thc Paleo movement needed to hear from a doctor in the trenches of conventional medicine who had used the principles to transform his own health and that of his patients. I had lost 130 pounds, significantly improved my health, and helped numerous patients avoid surgery, resolve chronic pain, and reclaim their lives. That, to me, was real medicine.

"*If one does not know to which port one is sailing, no wind is favorable.*"
—Lucius Annaeus Seneca, Rome, 65 AD

Dr. Jack Kruse

REFERENCES

1. http://www.theatlantic.com/magazine/archive/2010/11/lies-damned-lies-and-medical-science/8269/
2. http://www.scientificamerican.com/article.cfm?id=vitamins-minerals-and-microrna

Chapter One

CLOSING THE GREAT DIVIDE

"The saddest aspect of life right now is that science gathers knowledge faster than society gathers wisdom."
—Isaac Asimov

One of my favorite examples of the Epi-paleo Rx is Terry Wahls, M.D. and her story of re-engineering a broken body back to normalcy. It represents everything that is wrong in medicine today and is a story the world needs to hear.

Wahls is a family practice physician who was stricken with secondary progressive multiple sclerosis, an autoimmune disease my profession says has no cure. She became so sick she was relegated to a wheelchair as life slowly slipped from her grip. She initially entrusted her care to modern medicine, swimming in the same pool of knowledge as her doctors, except that now she was the patient and did not have the power she was accustomed to having. Our profession failed her miserably and she almost died. When she realized her fellow doctors had no answers, she turned to re-educating herself and to find light in the void of knowledge regarding her disease.

Her reading led her to the Paleo diet, a spark of light in the darkness. This spark lit a fuse that exploded into new truths, and she was able to cure her disease using her new "owner's manual." Instead of digging her own ditch deeper with conventional medicine, she threw away the shovel and thought about another way out of her nightmare.

Wahls' multiple sclerosis prompted her to question the medical dogma pounded into the heads of physicians. She abandoned conventional medicine for an educational crusade that healed her from a disease we were taught in medical school has no cure. Wahls found relying on pharmaceuticals to treat a sick person pales in comparison to relying on what evolution has honed for millions of years to shape our genes, body, and behavior. She learned that we have a biological wisdom hardwired[EF14] into us that tells us how we should eat to maintain optimal health, and that wisdom should be the cornerstone of all medical treatments.

WHAT IS THE EPI-PALEO RX?

If you spent $250,000 on a Rolls Royce, would you put cheap gas in it? If you bought a brand new laptop, would you load it with suboptimal software? Of course not, so why don't we treat our bodies, the most magnificent machine we'll ever operate in our lifetimes, the same way? Why do we expect optimal health when we eat a diet filled with processed and man-made foods? We live under artificial lights when it should be dark and we read books at night on LED screens that shoot signals to our retinas that the sun just rose and it's time to wake up and get going. We blast music into our ears priming us to run from a pride of big cats. People in Canada can now enjoy a banana in the dead of winter because our Neolithic brains have allowed us to overcome the biologic impossibility of bananas being available in Canada. Yet this amazing ability to alter our environment has become a detriment to our genome, which holds the entirety of our hereditary information, and we wonder why we face unprecedented Neolithic diseases today. We are capable of creating our environment to the detriment of our biology. We have this incredibly capable, evolving human brain wired into a Paleolithic body that has not caught up.

I failed for years to account for this biologic incongruence in myself and in my patients. The inspiration for this book comes from the regret I feel for failing my patients before this transforming insight, thanks to having been lost in the conventional mindset.

I eventually realized there was a basic truth I had denied too long. All living beings have an owner's manual that is not in any medical textbook but it is hardwired in their DNA by evolution. Our own evolutionary history is the ultimate reference book for optimal health. Sadly, my profession has never cracked that book to help a damn person.

As the medical scientist Peter Gluckman pointed out in his textbook Principles of Evolutionary Medicine, humans evolved an enlarged brain for the ability to form words to communicate. We can also create complex social networks and modern machinery. However, our largest contribution to evolution might be our ability to create a new reality with our thoughts. If these thoughts are mistaken, we can quickly recalculate and overcome the error of our mind. This attribute allowed humans to dramatically alter the ecosystems to which we are naturally adapted, and has set us on many new paths of evolution. Unfortunately, however, I believe the rapid rise of Neolithic diseases happens to be one of those paths. For all our evolutionary leaps forward, we are still prisoners of our paleocortex, the older, less-evolved brain that resists change and favors emotional whims and desires. The human conundrum is that often our habitual actions are driven by emotion instead of intellect.

We are mismatched to our current environment because of what our thoughts have created. We all know that when we eat badly we are making a decision that could ultimately kill us, albeit, slowly. I watch "serial suicide" daily at the fast-food drive-through joints and in the hospital cafeteria. Disease by food is insidious and sinister because the consequences are not apparent until the person ends up in an office like mine with a chronic health condition.

We need to abolish the paradox of our marvelous brain's capacity to alter our environment to the detriment of our ancestral genes. Moreover, we need to realize this mismatch is the Rosetta Stone to regaining optimal health.

My personal story is similar to Wahls', except I was not afflicted with a potentially lethal disease. I simply tore the meniscus in my knee when I stood up to give a talk on spine surgery. In that instant, all my primal instincts returned to me, and instead of thinking like a neurosurgeon, I listened to my primal sense. Wahls' situation was more desperate, and that desperation led her to challenge the dogma of conventional medicine.

Wahls has already crossed that threshold, both personally and professionally. Her story, my story, and your dissatisfaction with physicians need to be felt every day by organized medicine. This echo needs to resonate multiple times until they get the message that what we are teaching in medical school is missing the core element in healing. That missing link is treating human disease using an evolutionary paradigm to guide us.

WHY MEDICINE NEEDS AN AUTOPSY

I now scoff at my fellow MDs when they invoke the latest randomized control trial (RCT) data as proof for causation of anything. They laugh at me because they think I don't believe today's evidence-based medicine. Scientific data, very likely flawed and generated with money from those who stand to benefit from it, should trump two million years of an unbiased experiment in human life? My sensibilities are different now and I no longer jump to change my practice every time a new RCT comes out. There is a time and place for the benefits of RCT, but for too long we have ignored the dangers of relying predominantly on RCT data.

This is a problem for medicine. We lead the industrialized world in health care costs, yet rank last in life expectancy. This is insanity for a "super power" nation. We dispense a pill for every ill and have killed more than a quarter of a million people between 1976 and 2006 due to medication errors. You might think this fact alone would catch attention, but it has fallen on deaf ears.

I am not saying that we should ignore new RCT information. I am saying we first need to use what we already know to successfully treat Neolithic disease before we invoke the latest new implant or drug. We need to marry the best of both worlds to extract the full potential of what our species has to offer. How can 2 million years of nature's experiments not be good enough for modern health care?

Attack conventional medicine, and doctors often respond ferociously to protect their turf. Look at how cardiology defends the belief that saturated fats cause heart disease, despite lack of evidence. Patients will tell you they take statins, eat a low-fat, high-carbohydrate diet as prescribed by their doctors, and have very low cholesterol, yet still they succumb to heart disease, the number-one cause of death in men and women. This is how Albert Einstein defined insanity-doing the same thing over and over and expecting different results.

MEDICINE'S FAILING OF MODERN HUMANS

Here is one story of how modern science is failing us. On November 30, 2006, The CEO of Pfizer met with his research team in Groton, Connecticut to discuss their new blockbuster cholesterol drug torcetrapib. This drug, designed to raise HDL, was nearly through the gauntlet of phase-three clinical trials and close to getting FDA approval. Pfizer's main cholesterol-lowering drug, Lipitor, was due to come off patent soon and torcetrapib was their financial salvation. When a drug goes off patent the company loses its exclusivity to it, opening the door to generic versions that cost up to 80 percent less. As you can imagine, drug companies hate this. At the time, Lipitor was the most widely prescribed drug in the world, making Pfizer billions of dollars in profit. Kindler and researchers believed that if they could design a drug that raises HDL to be taken with Lipitor, which lowers LDL, they could win an even bigger share of the statin buffet.

Pfizer, their researchers, and most of organized medicine believe high cholesterol levels cause heart disease. However, cholesterol is an essential component of cell membranes, it makes up 70 percent of the structure of the human brain, and is the major building block for every steroid hormone the brain and body use. Cholesterol also patches areas of the blood vessels damaged by inflammation with small yellow plaques. That is how evolution designed this system.

It is true that elevated levels of oxidized cholesterol are associated with blockages of coronary and other major arteries. Cholesterol is the dynamite and the inflammation is the match. The foods that cause inflammation and oxidization are not found in abundance in nature. The modern diet, however, piles inflammatory foods onto our plates. Yet medicine ignores this and locks onto the theory of absolute cholesterol levels.

Lipitor works by lowering the low-density lipoprotein (LDL), commonly referred to as "bad" cholesterol. The major function of HDL is to transfer "bad LDL" back to the liver for recycling. HDL essentially renews old, used-up arterial patches. It clears them from the system so they don't fill up the arteries and block blood flow, causing heart attacks or strokes.

Torcetrapib works on an enzyme that recycles LDL back to HDL. Pfizer thought it could raise good cholesterol while lowering the bad LDL, thus making it an ideal way to treat heart disease. This, of course, assumes cholesterol determines heart disease. The drug was in the last stages of these clinical trials and Pfizer was so sure of its new blockbuster drug that it was ready to seek FDA approval to have it replace Lipitor. But something bad happened.

Evolutionary medicine rose up and bit him in the ass. During the last trials of the drug, patients taking torcetrapib with Lipitor experienced more cardiovascular problems and a 60 percent increase in death compared to patients taking Lipitor with a placebo. Pfizer immediately terminated the studies, which had cost $800 million. How could torcetrapib fail after all the hard science? Because lipids don't cause heart disease. Inflammation does. And diet above all else controls the inflammation in our serum. Altering the cholesterol pathways appears to be a great way to kill a person, because without cholesterol humans cannot live. Cholesterol is vital to many biochemical pathways forged by two million years of evolutionary testing.

This debacle shines light on what is wrong with our healthcare system today. It appears the system believes the more data scientists throw on top of a flawed hypothesis, the more believable it is. This gives pharmaceutical companies a tool for profit for which the government has no brake pedal, thanks to "scientific evidence" that is not independent science. The more shocking part of this story is that hundreds of scientists have known this hypothesis was total bullshit from the get-go. Uffe Ravnskov, MD, PhD is one of those men. He has written extensively about this issue yet no one bothered to have him sit on panels to review the science. In fact, a network of independent scientist who are cholesterol skeptics created the organization THINCS, which stands for The International Network of Cholesterol Skeptics.

I do not expect health care to get this message before you do. It's why Wahls and I had to solve our own problems. Medicine is incapable of helping us because it does not see the fallacy of its core principles. If it did, there would be thousands of articles questioning the lipid hypothesis in every major journal. Big pharma would go broke and CNBC would totally meltdown.

If scientists were correct with the lipid hypothesis, torcetrapib would have been spot on, yet it was a colossal failure. And now they are trying to validate torcetrapib in the journals with explanations that are plain insulting. It is clear they have learned nothing.

When I became aware of the truth, I began to challenge everything I believed. I suddenly recalled with laser precision the time in medical school in 1986 when a biochemistry professor warned me about the cholesterol hypothesis. It was my primal instinct texting my gut and I didn't listen. Next time, more than 20 years later, 130 pounds overweight, injured, and clearly failing so many of my patients, I listened.

Many resist a Paleolithic template because the diet requires you to eat everything we were taught in medical school would kill you. I can assure you the health of my family, many of my patients, and myself has improved significantly since we changed course to align with biologic truths.

Medicine's denial detracts from the real reasons why heart disease remains the number-one killer of men and women today. Doctors seem to enjoy blaming the patient's diet, accusing them of not complying with the very diet that causes heart disease. They constantly send you this message on the news, in the paper, in the magazines, and on the websites you read, especially if you're obese.

HOW A COVERT OMISSION CAN KILL YOUR HEART FASTER THAN A BIG MAC

Many doctors point to the success of the very low-fat Ornish diet, developed my Dean Ornish, MD, for heart health. Here is a case where a respected conventional medical doctor misrepresents data for his own ego. In a study on the diet, Ornish overlooks three other factors known to help reduce heart disease, and instead gives all the credit to his ultra-low-fat diet.

Mike Eades, MD, author of Protein Power, documents the fallacy of the Ornish diet. The science shows the Ornish diet increases inflammation and causes bacterial overgrowth in the small intestines. Moreover, Ornish's study is poorly designed due to a lack of proper controls, which confounded the four main variables in the study. The diet didn't reverse heart disease at all if you review the real data instead of the opinion of Ornish.

Eades wrote a blog post in 2006 that encapsulates why Ornish's claims are meaningless and continue to confuse many heart patients today. Here are some of Dr. Eades comments from that blog:

> *"After one year, 82% of the subjects in the treatment group (23 of 28) showed a regression (a very slight regression) of their coronary artery narrowing while those in the usual-care group showed a very slight increase in arterial narrowing. And subjects in the treatment group had fewer episodes of chest pain and other cardiac symptoms than their compatriots in the other group. Ignoring the most bogus part of this study, which is the fact that it is virtually impossible to determine the slight differences in arterial narrowing shown in this study and ignoring the fact that there were a number*

of patients "lost" to follow up in the treatment group (losing the right subjects can make data look a lot better statistically) and ignoring the fact that the randomization process wasn't exactly according to Hoyle and ignoring the fact that the only death in the study was in the treatment group, I still believe the subjects in the intervention group got better and probably did improve their coronary artery disease (I say this with one caveat that I'll address in a moment). I just don't believe they improved for the same reasons that Dr. Ornish does. If we look at how the study was structured, we see that the subjects were put on a lifestyle modification program.

In fact, the study was called 'The Lifestyle Heart Trial.' The subjects modified their lifestyles in four basic ways:

They went on a low-fat vegetarian diet

They stopped smoking

They began meditation and stress management

They started to exercise

We know that smoking is disastrous for people with coronary artery disease and that stopping smoking helps immeasurably. We know that exercise improves coronary blood flow and all around fitness and decreases mortality. And we suspect from the studies above mentioned in the Wall Street Journal article that meditation and stress reduction improves cardiac function and decreases cardiac mortality. If you have heart disease and you do these three things, odds are you're going to get better.

But what about the low-fat vegetarian diet? The low-fat diet by itself, unlike the other three activities, hasn't been shown conclusively to improve cardiac function. In fact, based on the recent accumulation of studies comparing low-fat diets to low-carbohydrate, higher fat diets, the low-fat diet has faired poorly. It is my opinion that the subjects in the Ornish study took three steps forward and one step back. The three steps forward, i.e., the smoking cessation, exercise, and meditation improved their cardiac function more than the low-fat diet they followed damaged it, leading to an overall improvement in their condition.

What evidence do I have to make that assertion? If you take a look at the lipid values of the subjects following the low-fat vegetarian diet you notice a fairly sinister finding (the caveat mentioned above): triglycerides went up markedly while HDL-cholesterol levels fell. Exactly the opposite of what you would like to see in patients with heart disease.

When this paper was published in 1990, the lipid focus was on total cholesterol and LDL-cholesterol, both of which fell in this study. Over the intervening years some pretty conclusive evidence has accumulated showing that if the lipid hypothesis of heart disease is valid-and Dr. Ornish certainly believes it is-then a rise in triglycerides and a fall in HDL are ominous signs, signs, in fact, that your therapy isn't working. If this study were published today, one wonders if the lipid values that looked so good to 1990 eyes would even be listed. (Happily, we who prescribe low-carbohydrate diets don't have to worry because triglycerides always fall and HDL usually goes up.)

Now getting to what agitates me about all this...I'm annoyed because Ornish, who never fails to mention that he has 'proven' that he can reverse heart disease, always attributes the improvement of the subjects in the treatment group to the low-fat diet they followed. Whenever anyone brings up the fact that it was a comprehensive program of lifestyle modification that did the trick (if the trick was really done), he always minimizes the role of the three activities known by everyone to improve vascular disease and emphasizes the role his diet played.

I believe that if this same study had been carried out using the same interventional modalities except that a low-carb diet had been substituted for the low-fat diet, the results would have been significantly better. The subjects in the treatment group would have taken four steps forward."

◇◇

Ornish is one reason people today still think a low-fat diet is good for your heart. While Ornish should be congratulated for linking mindfulness with lowering heart disease risk, he has caused immeasurable damage with a flawed diet that fosters mediocrity in our species.

CAN ONE OVERCOME A BAD DIET?

It is clear from the Paleolithic data there is no evidence of humans subsisting on a predominantly plant-based diet anywhere in the fossil record.

I ask my patients to ponder this, "If the medical profession was so correct about fats causing heart disease, how come after 50 years of a low-fat, high-carbohydrate diet and the liberal use of cholesterol lowering drugs, heart disease is still the number-one killer of men and women?"

Those who believe the lipid dogma will continue to find and fund studies that support it, no matter how flawed, as the system depends on their survival. The pharmaceutical and cardiology industries used a huge media campaign to explain away the disastrous results of the torcetrapib debacle so that they can continue to feed at the trough of cholesterol drug sales at your expense. Instead of listening to a panel of experts from the American Heart Association, American Diabetic Association, American Cardiology Association, or even the FDA, I want you to examine the data for yourself through the lens of human biology.

In my own practice, I do things very differently than how I was taught. I examine clinical issues using what I have learned about evolutionary medicine before jumping into a Neolithic "cure" with drugs or surgery. I also tell my patients my opinion-no more shades of grey blaming genetics or some other falsehood.

I often can predict what a patient's lab testing will reveal before I even order it, based on their history, their physical, and their MRI findings. Patients marvel at the accuracies when their labs come back. I explain to them that I am no smarter than my peers. I just now pay attention to things my peers were never taught that matter. I reassure them that most physicians work hard and do their best to be good doctors. I, however, no longer want to be a good doctor. I want to be a great doctor, and when I found out what evolutionary medicine could add to my medical toolbox, I jumped at the chance to use it. Evolution is the greatest medical textbook from which I have ever learned.

CONVENTIONAL WISDOM

Your primary health goal should be to avoid doctors and hospitals at all costs. Many times patients come to us feeling bad and we tell them they are fine, even when they know something is definitely wrong. That is primal instinct banging heads with conventional wisdom, and it is the source of so much patient distress. Doctors dismiss your complaint as genetic or stress and hand you a prescription for Prozac.

Many of my elderly patients tell me they spend more money on drugs than food. Drug companies offer humanitarian aid for these less fortunate folks, which is like applying a salve to a gaping wound. Most physicians applaud this noble show of grace. I think it is horseshit.

I write 90 percent fewer prescriptions today then I did five years ago after embarking on my Epi-paleo Rx journey. My patients are healthier and enjoy better outcomes from surgical procedures (should they still need them). They now enjoy the benefit of a surgeon who looks at their case through an evolutionary lens, an education that never stops growing. I want my poor and elderly patients to spend less money on drugs and more on food, as diet is the first step in transforming health, regardless of age or disability. You become your own physician by eating foods that match your evolutionary blueprint, thus controlling the cause of disease.

What we have today is a species in decline. We eat things created by mad scientists that then make us dependent on drugs for the illnesses they cause. If you allow my profession to tell you what to eat you may develop Neolithic diseases.

Don't waste your time blaming our government, medicine, and industrial agricultural. They are not going to change to suit your health care needs. The system was designed to make money off of sick people, not keep you well.

As a surgeon, health care embarrasses me. For every single patient I have failed while under the trance of conventional medicine, this book is my payback to you. Selfishly, I used it to fix myself first. I had to see if what I learned about Mother Nature had clinical effect.

Many of you on Internet forums and in clinics around the world have fueled my passionate, incendiary tone. A controlled rage now courses through my veins, and I want this information to spread across the globe as fast as possible. We don't need a stamp of approval from specialty boards of medicine before we give it to the masses. Thousands of people world-wide already live this template, and their results are testimony to the clinical greatness evolution has already hardwired into us.

I am actively recruiting medical doctors to help more of you. I am confident there are many physicians out there who sense we have had much of it wrong. Patient and doctor are equals now-we share the same owners manual, regardless of how much more education or knowledge a doctor might have. Anyway, most people do not care how much you know until they know how much you care.

I hope you can forgive the medical profession for the mistakes we have made at your expense. I can assure you we did not do it on purpose. We became intellectually lazy and stopped following the same biological blueprint that works for every other animal on this planet. Animals do not have a Neolithic brain that allows them to outpace their DNA.

My sphere of influence in my community is small. Real change is difficult for physicians as the system penalizes us for stepping out of line. If a physician does not write a prescription for a statin drug for a certain cholesterol level, it affects their reimbursement by insurance. Many times the health care system dictates the actions of your doctors; their hands are tied. The power to practice medicine has been stripped from the people who have the knowledge to help you most. The system is set up to keep you sick. But you can thank your doctor for trying to help you, fold that statin prescription in half, place it in a drawer, and not fill it. You will know when your doctor is on your team when they hand you the prescription with a wink.

PRIMAL IMPACT

We Neolithic humans have shown ourselves adept at altering our environment, why not change the medical paradigm? Each person's health transformation can have global effects. The revolution that will save the world is ultimately a personal one. It's time for that battle to be fought.

You-my patients, my readers, and those of you in the Paleo community-have opened my eyes. Thanks for insight folks, and for getting me back on the evolutionary track. Find pleasure in primal chaos. It might save your life. Just ask Dr. Terry Wahls.

REFERENCES

1. http://www.nytimes.com/2010/09/16/health/16chen.html?src=tp&smid=fb-share
2. http://paleodietnews.com/3803/paleo-diet-why-doctors-know-nothing-about-nutrition/
3. http://journals.lww.com/academicmedicine/Abstract/2010/09000/Nutrition_Education_in_U_S__Medical_Schools_.30.aspx
4. http://www.citizen.org/documents/rapidlyincreasingcriminalandcivilpenalties.pdf
5. http://www.proteinpower.com/drmike/cardiovascular-disease/three-steps-forward/

Chapter Two

PRIMAL SENSE: IT COMES WITH YOUR BIOLOGY, SO USE IT.

"Failure is the condiment that gives success its flavor."
–Truman Capote

Sharing my vision of what healthcare should become excites many of my patients yet disconcerts others as this new paradigm involves no handholding. It requires you, the patient, to think like an evolutionary adventurer exploring your own physiology.

One of my patients, Lynn, talked about the patient's role in transforming the paradigm of medicine: "I changed doctors because my first doctor was impatient with me, and pushing statins on me. I refused them. It was an example of my getting enough courage to take responsibility for my health, which felt good."

Your gut is often your best early warning system. If what you're told in our offices does not sound right, do not accept it. The public today thinks, "Well, the doctor must know more than me, as I have no formal training." That train of thought might kill you. It almost killed Wahls until she relied on her primal instinct to find a real answer.

A doctor will know more than the patient about conventional medicine, but a patient can educate herself on how to stay healthy and even run her own labs. Books such as The Primal Blueprint, The Paleo Solution, The Perfect Health Diet, Primal Body, Primal Mind, Life Without Bread, and The New Evolutionary Diet explain which foods keep us healthy and disease-free. The amount of science behind these books is impressive if you read their references. They are certainly better researched than the USDA diet most dietitians and nutritionists recommend.

The USDA diet is designed to do one thing only-make money for those who sell it to the rest of the world. Most people, including dietitians and nutritionists, don't realize industrial food giants subsidize their educations. Medicine abdicated its responsibility to teach nutrition to the dieticians and nutritionists in the mid-20th century, an error that still impacts our health today. These professionals promote grains as a healthy choice, even though the science on the dangers of grains paints a totally different picture than the science funded by food corporations. People such as Loren Cordain, Ph.D. and paleoanthropologists all over the world have come to the same conclusions-the dawn of agriculture might be the biggest Neolithic error mankind has ever made. Its dominance is behind many of the diseases we see today. If you think this is hyperbole, read Wheat Belly by William Davis, MD. Even if Davis' critics are correct and half of his book is exaggerated, his book helps tear down the wall of misinformation that industrial agriculture has constructed to profit from their products. Eating grains consistently throughout your life will raise your risk of succumbing to many chronic Neolithic diseases our ancestors never experienced. The health of a grain-based diet is supported not by science but instead by dietitians educated by the corporate food giants, which are, in turn, backed by the government.

This book is not designed to discuss the merits of evolutionary medicine, but instead is a handbook is designed to give you the Epi-paleo Rx for the top diseases our species faces today. It isn't genes alone that determine our health destiny, but instead it's our food and lifestyle choices. Genes do not control us, they respond to what we do!

PRIMAL TOOLS IN THE MODERN ERA

We have the power of technology to help us create the state of optimal health. Electronic monitors, iPad and iPhone apps, and Internet point calculators can quantify our health. You can run your own lab tests to see how food affects your cells, and then make choices based on that information. I believe one day doctors will write prescriptions for iPhone apps instead of drugs.

SIRI and WATSON, the giant super computers from IBM, answer medical questions through a connection with the computing cloud, where information on the primal lifestyle is found. This kind of artificial intelligence (AI) is something our Paleolithic genes need to survive medicine today, especially in poor rural areas where people need the Epi-paleo Rx most.What if a handheld device could transport X-ray images from a West Virginia's coal mining town or a Laredo, Texas ghetto directly to the cloud for a second opinion using a Epi-paleo Rx lens? With a click we could tell the person the Big Macs they are eating are replacing marrow with fat, and that osteoporosis is an issue.

We could photograph a picture of acne or eczema and get a primal treatment plan immediately. The cloud would inform us that most skin diseases are surface manifestations of leaky gut, a condition in which the lining of the intestines become damaged and overly porous due to inflammation, and undigested foods and pathogens escape into the bloodstream to create more inflammation. Today, it seems no dermatologist is aware of this fact, but cloud computing could reveal the truth. Your skin moles could be sent to the cloud to determine whether they should be biopsied. So could your brain MRI, mammograms, and thyroid ultrasounds.

Many will scoff and say that there is no way this platform can handle such big data crunches. Let me introduce you to 23andMe genetic testing. Ten years ago it cost $1 billion to sequence your entire genome to reveal your single nucleotide polymorphisms (SNP), which determine your genetic risks for disease. Today, 23andMe can give you the same information for $99. If you sign up online, 23andMe emails you updates about your risks as science makes new discoveries. In 2011, 23andMe had 10,000 subscribers, although my bet is that figure will one day reach 10 million. Also, the genetic data we generate on these people will benefit mankind enormously, allowing us to analyze the effects of diet on biology. Can you imagine putting the data of millions of people into the cloud to analyze trends and escape allopathic medicine's belief systems? This information could one day allow science to prescribe a custom diet and targeted nutraceuticals or pharmaceuticals based on your DNA and genomic epitope.

Three-dimensional scanning and printing is already a health care trend. For instance, a three-dimensional scan can scan the leg of a patient who lost the other leg in an accident. It can then build a prosthetic leg with matching skin tone and size. Three-dimensional printing is also integrating with stem cell research and regenerative medicine. It may one day be possible to create libraries of replacement tissues and perhaps even organs.

Another example is the effect of online social networks on our behavior. When your wireless scale shares your weight with your friends, you receive praise for success or pressure to maintain your diet. Social networks are also powerful tools to track and predict disease. James Fowler, co-author of the book Connected, is working with Facebook to look at health data. For example, the more friends you have, the earlier in the flu season you'll get influenza. Their work could help predict when you'll get the flu steps to take to avoid it. People also can share their medical histories, treatment failures, and success stories through such platforms as PatientsLikeMe.com and CureTogether.com.

Genomera.com crowd-sources health data from individuals to better understand health. Practice Fusion crowd-sources data from electronic medical records. By collecting data from all patients within a hospital or a region, you can see trends and run clinical studies on the fly. For example, you could see all the patients with a certain gene taking the same drug, and determine if that drug is effective.

I already communicate with patients over Webex and Skype. I believe one day this is how I will see 99 percent of my patients. AliveCor made an iPhone app to transmit ECGs from your phone to my computer. This way, you don't need to come in to see us for chest pain if we can see from your ECG that everything is OK. We also can do the same for diabetics and their blood sugar levels. Others are turning iPhones into otoscopes to look in their child's ear and send the info via the cloud to the doctor. These are but a few examples of how Neolithic thought synchronizes with our biologic directives. Embrace these changes and become part of them, for you will change medicine while most doctors are still asleep at the wheel writing prescriptions for a statin.

These advances in technology allow us to personalize medicine. For example, we can customize cancer chemotherapy based on tumor types and their genomic expressions. We can measure heart rates and exercises parameters, and check the nutrition density of our diet by using a cell phone application. If you get a regular lipid panel that does not have the necessary markers on it, you can add it through a website. You can order a salivary or serum hormone test on your own if your doctor does not want to order it for you.

You can then bring these lab results to your doctor and share in the decision-making process. Your doctor may not know what the new labs mean, but he or she may know someone who does and who can help you. By using these lab tests to shine a light on possible underlying causes to your condition, it forces the health care professional to alter the treatment plan based on the new data. The doctor is medically and legally required to integrate this new data into a treatment plan. This is not widely known or talked about, but introducing new data can help you avoid cookie-cutter treatment plans.

For example, we discovered during surgery that one of my patients had osteoporosis, as her bone would not hold the screws well due to poor mineral content. At a follow-up appointment, I told her a gynecologist needed to evaluate her hormone status. Because she was younger and still menstruating, I knew the gynecologist would resist working up her problem. So I told her how to ask for what she wanted based upon the testing we already had done. I also told her that the osteoporosis might be caused by a leaky gut stemming from possible celiac disease, and that she also needed a work up by a gastroenterologist. I told her how to ask the right questions to get these doctors to order the correct tests. I warned her the doctors might not be open to the message she was bringing, but that should not deter her. She encountered exactly what I expected, but she persisted and was able to navigate the process by knowing what to ask. She got to the bottom of her problem, changed the course of her disease, and ultimately the course of her life.

The more data a patient has the more information she can give the doctor. Physicians are taught to respond to numbers, so I say give them more numbers if you want to transform your relationship with them. The most common complaint I hear from patients these days is, "My doctor does not listen to me." Create the doctor you want by helping them help you.

It turned out my neck-fusion patient had severe hormonal disruption and a gastrointestinal disorder. She was able to make her care useful by getting as much testing as possible. She does this routinely now, and always comes in with stories about how she helps direct her own care. She is empowered, and very happy about it.

PATIENTS NEED TO SEE TO BELIEVE

The reason many people and doctors are unaware of the effect diet has on health is because the effects are not always immediately obvious. About 80 percent of human learning comes from visual inputs. If we can't see it, we don't know it exists. Also, as health deteriorates the brain cannot make the necessary chemicals to think well, so you further lose the ability to see the less obvious truths and make good choices. I see this in my patients with Alzheimer's disease, a disease exploding across all demographics. This is no longer a geriatric disease, but a nutritional disease, a fact medicine and government seem to ignore despite epidemiology data. Most people think it's a normal part of getting older, but it's 100 percent preventable.

When someone looks at a book about elderly hunter-gatherers and sees what 70 years old is supposed to look like, they are shocked at what they see in themselves. This is how a human learns best. Showing someone what to do is more important than telling someone, because our brain works best with something visual. This is an easy change we can implement to help those who cannot help themselves.

I now show my spine patients what an older hunter-gatherer looks like and what they accomplish in a day. YouTube also allows them to do this. Most of my older patients can barely walk to the mailbox, and some urinate without control. I have 50-year-old patients who need to wear a diaper. I tell them this is not normal human aging, this is what you get when you are socialized to believe the SAD is OK because everyone else does it. Taking 18 different prescription drugs in your later years is not normal. We are not on this planet to become medical annuities for medicine.

When showing patients the evidence does not work, I ask them to tell me their favorite comfort food. Inevitably it contains wheat. I then share with them a few thoughts from the book Wheat Belly. When people learn how badly grains affect human health, it dismantles some of their socialized beliefs. When people at church talk to me about grains, they ask, "Then why does my doctor say they are so good?" I simply refer them to the book Life Without Bread and tell them to Google "grains and disease." The thousands of references astound them, and they want to know, "Why isn't anyone talking about this?"

I don't treat society in my office, I treat patients, and my duty is to open their eyes and their minds to what really ails them. When they commit to change, I then work my hardest to help them get where they want to be. Many people think that just because we have been eating bread for 10,000 years it's OK. However, science can have a way of making even the most hardcore processed-food addicts come around eventually. If not, they eventually wind up on an operating table with a Neolithic disease. In my clinic, I give them the choice between the status quo or a new way to live, and if they're willing to change I tell them how I did it and how I have helped hundreds of others do it during the last five years.

Health is not just about which foods you eat and exercises you perform; it's also about how well you are able to control how you think. I personally believe that controlling the way you think is the first and most important step in the Epi-paleo Rx of health. I view a thought like an endocrinologist views a dose of growth hormone. Both are secreted from the brain, and both exert a targeted biologic effect. One thought is capable of changing everything in your life.

REFERENCES

1. http://techcrunch.com/2012/01/01/healthtech-2012/
2. http://www.ajconline.org/article/S0002-9149(11)02748-2/abstract

CHAPTER THREE

USING PRIMAL SENSE TO ADAPT TO CHANGE

HOW DO WE TRANSFORM THOUGHT TO EVOLVE?

Your health is tied to your chronic modes of thinking. How do you get out of a thinking rut? How do you embrace change when your heart or your will is broken? How do you re-engineer a life? I get asked this a lot. Instead of answering it directly, I tell people to listen to how I say the words I believe to be truths. Listen to the passion in my voice and the cadence of my speech. None of it is contrived. Passion cannot be faked or bought. When authenticity is perceived as genuine, our gut senses it before our brain does. Carl Jung once said, "Until you make the unconscious conscious, it will direct your life and you will call it fate."

The first change you must make in the Epi-paleo Rx is to control how you think and trust your vision when no one else does. If you don't believe in what you're doing people will perceive thatbefore you even complete your thoughts or actions. People don't care what you know until they know how much you care.

I am now intolerant of mediocrity. Society rewards mediocrity. Every child gets a trophy. Can you imagine the swamp we would still be in if evolution followed the same logic? No matter the poor choices I have made, I am never too old, too bad, too late, or too sick to start from scratch again.

Christopher Columbus said we cannot discover new oceans unless we have the courage to lose sight of the shoreline. We must embrace our worse fears to do so. Failure teaches us right from wrong in most things. In surgery if you fail too often you will quickly be out of business. I had to learn to avoid errors early in my training through good preparation and by reading about other's failures. However, avoiding failure set me back personally.

Also, the stress never stops, so you must learn how to adapt or it will eventually kill you. It is the fuel that powers evolution. That was my epiphany that I had to "get out of line" and start anew. You must constantly adapt to life or you will die unhappy.

Remembering you are going to die one day is the best way to avoid thinking you have something to lose. There is absolutely no reason not to follow your heart or your passion here and now. If what you're doing in life is not your passion, then you have nothing to lose by changing right now.

Nothing diminishes anxiety faster than action. Action is always a better choice than inaction. The best thing you can do is the right thing; the next best thing you can do is the wrong thing; the worst thing you can do is nothing. Evolution punishes inaction. As a surgeon, seeing death daily made me realize the greatest mistake we can make is to live in constant fear of making an error. I can accept failure but I can't accept not trying my best.

Eighty percent of the information we get from life comes through our visual inputs. But what we see with our eyes pales in comparison to what we see with our thoughts via our mind's eye. This is the realm where our creative being lives and can imagine what we can become. I visit this place every morning when the sun rises and open my perception to a new reality. This was core part to my Epi-paleo Rx.

Today, consider opening your heart and mind to the wonders around you. Let this awareness flow through you and touch your mind. Let gratitude for life's daily blessings overflow inside you. Swim in the "new you" for a time. This is how a thought can change your DNA, and how happiness revealed itself to me five years ago. You are the captain of your ship and you must take control of the rudder to get where you want to go.

A PATIENT'S THOUGHTS

I want to share with you some of comments from my patient Jodi, a 40-year-old mother of three and former skeptic who completely transformed her body. I gave her a rough draft of this work early on and her reply touched me.

Jodi said, "I was reading your draft and thinking of all the different excuses I hear from my current friends who want to get my results but don't BELIEVE they're capable of making lifelong changes. I hear, 'I can't give up grains, so I'll just keep doing what I'm doing and maybe cut back on sweets.' Or they say, 'That's not a realistic lifestyle for a human.' Or they drop this bomb, 'You should do things in moderation, not go to such extremes. It's just not practical.' Or, my obese family member who says, 'I can't,' to just about every suggestion thrown at her.

I think once you cross that BELIEF barrier in your mind, you can do anything you want to. And with me, it took YOU to make me believe it was possible. It was like you getting in my face (well, cyberistically speaking) and saying, if you do what I tell you, you will have the body and health you never dreamed possible. I believed it. And so I did it." For those of you that have not seen the video yet, I operated on Jodi in 2007 for a neck fusion that caused spinal cord compression and could have paralyzed her. During her transformation, the only contact we had was through Facebook and the phone. I never once laid a hand on her during her transformation. Thoughts, however, radically changed her DNA as you will see.

She went on to say, "It's all about believing you have the ability to change your circumstances. Most people are unhappy with themselves but they wallow in their mediocrity because they don't feel they are strong enough, smart enough, or self-disciplined enough to change direction. It's sad, because like you said, fast forward 20-30 years, what will you look back on this time in your life and wish you could've done differently?

"Life really is too short to not take control of the things you truly CAN control, like what you eat and how much exercise you fit in your schedule. To me, this Paleolithic lifestyle and my exercise regime gives me a sense of control in a life that is often chaotic. No one can force a person to be unhealthy. Only we can do that to ourselves. It's all in your mind. And the mind is more powerful than we all think."

My parting thoughts in this chapter are inspired by a person who became the change he wanted to see . Ghandi said, "Man often becomes what he believes himself to be. If I keep on saying to myself that I cannot do a certain thing, it is possible that I may end by really becoming incapable of doing it. On the contrary, if I have the belief that I can do it, I shall surely acquire the capacity to do it even if I may not have it at the beginning."

You must transform your thoughts to transform your life. From that point forward, this transformation leads you to new paths you formerly could not imagine. This is the creative process in the right hemisphere of the brain that separates us from all other animals. It is a wonderful evolutionary asset if used properly, but it can also be the seat of our destruction if we allow Neolithic choices to override our Paleolithic blueprint.

The goal of the Epi-paleo Rx is to teach you how to master your Neolithic mind to protect your Paleolithic genes. I hope you remember this one thing: the Epi-paleo Rx is a directive for self-awareness. Stop letting convenience create dietary incompetency and poor health. This is why small lifestyle changes over time can lead to massive transformations on every level of our existence. We need to get in the habit of creating small "wins" to for big transformations.

REFERENCES

1. The Last Word on Power by Tracy Goss.
2. http://www.sebringclinic.com/documentation/HealthyHuman.pdf
3. Nesse RM, Stearns SC. The great opportunity: evolutionary applications to medicine and public health. Evol Appl2008;1:28-48.
4. AAMC-HHMI Scientific Foundation for Future Physicians Committee. Scientific foundations for future physicians. American Association of Medical Colleges and Howard Hughes Medical Institute, 2009.

Chapter Four

THE FUELS OF THE EPI-PALEO RX AND THE CURRENT POLICY OF TRUTH IN HEALTHCARE

THE POLICY OF TRUTH

Manuel Lora made this remark on my Facebook wall about the costs of food, "I love shattering the myth that people eat junk or processed food because it is cheaper. They eat this crap because they consider their health and quality of life to be a low priority compared to other mindless amusement and activities, such as online shopping, reality TV shows, and video gaming."

Poor thoughts begin with poor foods. If we eat nutrient-dense foods we can make superior neurochemicals in our brain that allow us to think like a genius. However, it seems our brain does not make this connection and it is why our species has become mediocre. Food companies have convinced us ketchup is a vegetable and zombie dietitians and nutritionists, who were educated by the USDA, reinforce the Neolithic belief that processed food is the same as real food. It is pure insanity to listen to these people and it is why our people are mediocre and dying a slow, painful, and expensive death.

In the early half of the 20th century, physicians wrote dietary prescriptions for certain diseases. That ended in the 1950s and 1960s when medicine allowed dietitians and nutritionists to usurp this process. The federal government set nutritional policy by subsidizing their education. Then in the 1970s, the federal government began making dietary policy political. Today, to graduate from one of these programs, you are force fed USDA dogma.

Nutritional therapy was a key feature in medical training in the early half of the 20th century. Between 1910 and 1945, the Columbia Presbyterian Hospital in New York City offered more than 50 unique therapeutic diets for diseases, following Hippocrates' advice to "let food be your medicine." Columbia University was not unique-this was typical of any major community or university hospital at that time. I trained at Charity Hospital In New Orleans, which was in operation for more than 150 years before Hurricane Katrina took it out in 2005. I remember going into the archives of the hospital as a resident and finding that the hospital offered six tubercular diets, four kidney diets, and eight gastrointestinal diets as late as the 1970s. Today, we believe there is no longer a need for dietary treatment because drugs have replaced them. I read about all the diets available for peptic ulcers up until 1988, when things moved to a pharmaceutical model alone.

Some see this as advancement. I see it as failure because we have not seen a declining disease rate using this paradigm. In fact, we have seen diseases of the gastrointestinal tract explode in the last 25 years since drugs were introduced as gold-standard therapies. Most other organ system diseases have seen the same rise.

Today it is considered a breach of the standard of care to question medical dogma. Doctors who question the dogma are ostracized and often the target of hostile acts by hospital administration and their peers, or banished from the hospital regardless of their clinical expertise and results. Playing ball with the system is paramount for survival. I faced this issue in my own hospital on trumped-up charges. A group of physicians who knew precisely what the system was capable of doing when you stepped out of line rescued me. It is hard to be a true advocate for patients today and not get in hot water with the system. In the last 20 years, to make sure they have total control over physicians, hospitals use medical staff committees to pass rules to punish doctors who step out of line. Most doctors cower to this abuse of power. Some of us fight back. Many times, their policies are direct attacks on patients' best interests and aligned with profit motives. They will see to it that the PR department interfaces with the local papers' health reporters to publish positive articles on their business practices.

Modern healthcare is phenomenal at treating acute medical problems, such as an epidural hematoma or a fractured leg or arm. But what we really suck at is treating chronic illness. And most of health care dollars are spent treating chronic health issues because our population eats a diet that fosters Neolithic disease. If we eat and live well, we should not require hospitalization. If and when it is needed, you should be the purveyor of when it is needed and why. You should not leave that up to anyone else. I know this sounds radical, but I promise you it is sound advice.

Did we learn anything from the history of 20th century medicine? In my opinion, the advent of vaccines, antibiotics, and public sanitation were noble efforts that made a difference in that era (although I realize vaccines are a controversial issue). So why do we rank so low in health care and mortality compared to our peers today? What the hell happened to health care in the 20th century? Costs rose while outcomes became exponentially worse.

It's called the introduction of business to medicine. On one hand, without the infusion of money by big business into medicine, many advances would have died on the vine. But the corollary is that many of the things that we had right were changed to suit business interests. We saw the emergence of major corporations in medical supplies and the direction of patient care by pharmaceutical companies. No one explains this to patients today, we just continue to spend billions treating symptoms that never eradicate any disease, and few ask why.

REFERENCES

1. Nesse RM, Williams GC. Why we get sick: the new science of Darwinian medicine. Times Books, 1995.
2. Stearns SC, Koella JC, editors. Evolution in health and disease. Oxford University Press, 2008.
3. Nesse RM, Stearns SC. The great opportunity: evolutionary applications to medicine and public health. Evol Appl2008;1:28-48
4. Gluckman PD, Beedle AS, Hanson MA. Principles of evolutionary medicine. Oxford University Press, 2009.

Chapter Five

WHAT ARE THE EPI-PALEO RX LAB PANEL TECHNIQUES TO BIO HACK ONE'S SELF?

How do you regain power over your health? You have to learn how to hack yourself-it's not that hard. Medical school didn't teach me about the labs I use, so I had to teach myself. If I can do it, so can you.

Since doctors use lab data to treat disease, you need to learn how to play in that sand box. The 16 lab tests below are the ones that I use most frequently in my own clinic. They are by no means the only ones. I want to discuss them here because I will mention them in coming chapters.

DR. KRUSE'S TOP 12 LAB TESTS

1. VO2 Max assessment (cardiopulmonary findings lead to a work up if needed)

A VO2 max, which measures maximal oxygen uptake, is now an easy test to get at many gyms. People with cardiovascular disease should seriously consider this test to know how much life is left in their lungs and heart. You can also use this bad boy to know how much high-intensity interval training (HIIT) you should start with. These are baselines and not set in stone.

A. VO2 max < 20 ml/kg/min: You should walk 15 min 5-7 days per week only.

B. VO2 max < 20-25 ml/kg/min: You should perform 15 minutes of aerobic work 5-7 days a week with one anaerobic interval. An anaerobic interval = 0-5 sec.

C. VO2 max < 25-30 ml/kg/min: You should perform 20 minutes of aerobic activity with 2 anaerobic Intervals 4-5 times a week. An interval = 5-15 sec

D. VO2 max < 30-35 ml/kg/min: You should perform 20 min of HIIT 4 times per week with 4 intervals. An interval is 5-5 sec.

E. VO2 max < 35-40 ml/kg/min: You should perform 20 minutes of HIIT 3 times a week with 4 intervals. An interval is 15-30 sec; recovery is 3-5 sec. You can also add 30 minutes of steady state cardio (sprints) once a week.

F. VO2 max <40-45 ml/kg/min: You should perform 20 minutes of HIIT 3 times a week with 5 or more intervals 3 days a week. An intervals can be greater than 30 sec. Recovery can be 1-2 minutes.

G. VO2 max 45+ ml/kg/min: You should perform 20 min of HIIT with 6 intervals 3 days a week. The interval is greater than 45 sec and your recovery must be less than 1 minute.

Note: One should only use the cold thermogenesis protocol if your VO2max is 25ml/kg/min.

2. DEXA body composition scan

Everyone should know his or her body composition. The standard body mass index (BMI) calculations and measurements are worthless, so I do not use them. The DEXA body scan gives you tremendous insight into what you are doing right and wrong, and how changes affect your body composition over time. If you do not care what your body is doing then skip it. For follow-up visits, I sometimes use bioimpedance assessments to limit radiation exposure from serial DEXA scanning. I fully expect major technological advancements to hit this area of testing.

3. Annual neuro-cognitive tests to assess processing speed, response speed, memory, learning, and attention

I use these tests to assess function of the brain, the body's ultimate organ. It tells us about the four main neurotransmitters and how they are working in unison. If one has depression, autism, or obsessive-compulsive disorder (OCD), it often means something is amiss with the building blocks of the brain. I no longer blame this on a genetic pre-disposition. Instead, a major hormonal problem involving progesterone, DHEA, or cortisol is usually behind it at some level. DHEA is the major hormone found in the young healthy brain. The hormones that drop like a Led Zeppelin as we pass the age of 35 are pregnenolone, progesterone, and DHEA. You can order these labs if your doctor won't, and they can be blood or saliva tests. Sometimes this test will lead me to run a micronutrition panel, like the one you can order online from SpectraCell (http://www.spectracell.com/). I love looking at intracellular glutathione often.

4. Comprehensive blood chemistry panel (Chem-20)

This is a good, straight-forward lab test of basic body chemistry. It is useful when you look at in the context of other variables. None of these labs dictate absolute treatment unless you have panic values, which I doubt most of you will have.

5. Liver function testing

6. Serum Iron, TIBC, Serum Ferritin and Iron % Saturation

These are straight-forward tests that are helpful for thyroid and anemia hacks. There is nothing special here. One can use a site like www.stopthethyroidmadness.com to help your own hack. I send my own patients there to learn what they need to know.

7. Lipid panels, such as VAP and/or NMR analysis

This is one is a biggie. I am going to go into some big-time detail here. When most people get a VAP they think heart, cholesterol and lipid study. I do not. I use this test to assess the brain-gut axis. You won't find this axis discussed in any allopathic textbook because they don't know yet that it exists.

Every medical doctor knows about asterixis. Asterixis is also called the flapping tremor, or liver flap. It is a tremor of the wrist when the wrist is extended, and is characterized by jerking movements of a patient's outstretched hands. Few doctors understand why it happens. It occurs because the liver is the brain's main protection from inflammation and environmental toxins. This is an area of the Epi-paleo Rx where you have a distinct advantage over your doctor. They will look at your lipid panel and think "heart disease risk." But you can look at it to see how successfully your liver's filtering abilities are managing inflammation, something you can control with diet, supplement changes, or further lifestyle alterations.

Most people in the primal world associate leaky gut with a gluten intolerance, however many things cause leaky gut, which I have written about on my blog. The VAP test is good for assessing gut function based on the fuels we are feeding it. If you dissect your VAP you can learn plenty about what you should and shouldn't be eating based upon your current cellular homeostasis. Most people think a diet is static, but if you are working to reverse a Neolithic disease, your diet should change according to your needs, which you can assess with testing. If you are already healthy but want optimal body composition, you just need to follow a Paleolithic diet outlined in the diet books I already mentioned. I personally use a quarterly lab draw system to assess my own health and make changes as necessary.

I think the real defender of gut integrity is not the brush border of the intestine but rather the liver's ability to detoxify our blood and ensure our plasma is not oxidized. The first line of defense after food is eaten is the gut-associated lymphoid tissue (GALT), also known as the gut's immune system. The foods we eat subject us to inflammation, as eating is the most common way our bodies interact with the environment-the more inflammatory the diet, the higher the risk of disease. The nutrients the gut absorbs enter the liver's portal circulation for detoxification and repackaging. This is the most important step in biology in my view. If the liver is a "poor sieve," you are opening the floodgates to inflammation and eventually Neolithic disease. So what allows the liver to be a good sieve? The answer is HDL, optimal testosterone and estrogen levels, good thyroid hormone levels, and a well functioning LDL receptor.

A healthy liver protects the gut and brain from assault. Most endotoxins (toxins in bacteria) gain access to our portal circulation but rarely make it to our general circulation, where they would cause real damage, because our liver won't allow it. In fact, the liver's ability to bind to endotoxins is increased by exercise, testosterone, estrogen, and even occasional alcohol use. This is why the occasional glass of red wine has benefited so many cultures over the eons. Excessive use, however, is not part of the Epi-paleo Rx because it disrupts the filtering capability of the liver.

A high HDL is a sign of good liver function. HDL particles bind to inflammatory endotoxin particles to protect us from oxidation. This is why a high HDL level confers general health and well being across the board. This has been repeatedly shown in many scientific journal articles and makes good primal sense, too. Moreover, very low-density lipoprotein (VLDL) and chylomicrons also protect us from inflammatory damage. This biologic process is at the seat of why we see higher cholesterol levels in the face of cellular stress or infection. Cholesterol production is our body's natural response to clean up inflammation if the brush border is overwhelmed in a situation of gut damage. We also need to be mindful that any stressor can increase the permeability of the gut, including cortisol, malabsorption, or infections.

Thyroid hormones back up liver function. If your gut receives an insult that causes leaky gut, thyroid hormone production increases to up-regulate turnover of cholesterol, working with vitamin A to convert cholesterol to pregnenolone. Pregnenolone is the basic building block of all the steroid hormones our brain uses to run the body. You may now begin to understand why I believe lowering your cholesterol makes zero sense from a biologic standpoint. Its formation is critical for our brain to manage the stress of many different cellular insults.

If this system is not working properly the result is a communication breakdown between the brain and our cells. This is how I globally define leptin resistance. Leptin resistance prohibits the brain from understanding a situation in the liver or elsewhere in the body. Likewise, when we lose control of our thyroid hormone production (hypothyroidism) we essentially lose control of the brain's communication with peripheral cells. Also, we can no longer effectively make steroid hormones from pregnenolone. When cortisol is chronically elevated, the body steals pregnenolone from the other hormones to make cortisol, decreasing progesterone, DHEA, estrogen, testosterone, and vitamin D. This helps explain why we see low vitamin D, testosterone, and estrogen in so many people today. Life today is based on a constant need for cortisol due to our inflammatory diets, our unnatural exposure to light late into the night, and other Neolithic factors.

So we need to think about the thyroid some more. Here is another biochemical fact few realize: 20 percent of the conversion of T4 to T3 (this is the conversion of inactive thyroid hormone to active thyroid hormone our body can use, hence a vital process) occurs directly in the gut. The liver primarily converts the remainder. So the liver and thyroid is critical to how this brain gut axis system works.

If the brain senses thyroid hormones are low it increases the secretion of thyroid-stimulating hormone (TSH) from the pituitary gland. This increased secretion is pro-inflammatory as it causes the liver to make a chemical called high-sensitivity C-reactive protein (HS-CRP). HS-CRP is a chemical that is what we call an acute phase reactant. This means the liver releases it whenever we face any kind of metabolic stress. The same is true for ferritin, which is stored in the reticuloendothelial system of the liver. There are other acute phase reactants but these two are the most important.

HS-CRP, which is not the same as CRP, is what we used to measure baseline inflammation in patients. This is a lab I order all the time in my clinic, and one you need to follow closely as you age. It is a relatively new test in medicine that most cardiologists use. HS-CRP tells you how oxidized your plasma is, which in turn tells you how much inflammation your cells are making in response to you food and your environment. You want HS-CRP as close to zero as possible. Inflammation underpins your risk for most Neolithic diseases.

High CRP levels are known to walk hand in hand with the development of heart disease, atherosclerosis, many brain diseases, and many autoimmune diseases. As HS-CRP made in the liver multiplies, it facilitates the production of pro-inflammatory chemicals called cytokines. Cytokines stimulate inflammation, including in the blood vessels, which provokes the rupture of plaques. This is why 55 percent of fatal heart attacks are caused by plaque rupture instead of arterial occlusion. When your HS-CRP is elevated you better take notice; it is a great way to globally assess inflammatory risk.

Hypothyroidism is correlated with heart disease and many autoimmune conditions. Hashimoto's thyroiditis is an epidemic in America and in my view is a sign of a constant assault on the gut that eventually floods liver portal circulation with inflammation.

This is a simplified version of the physiology of the brain-gut axis. Once inflammatory cytokines are present in the general circulation they head to the two most prominent organs based upon blood flow-the brain and the heart. The first effect in the brain is to overwhelm the parts not protected by the blood-brain barrier, which are also the areas that secrete hormones in response to both the external and internal environments.

The most important of these unprotected areas are found in the hypothalamus, where the leptin receptors are also located. These receptors can become so overwhelmed by inflammatory cytokines that they become resistant. Leptin resistance, in turn, basically blinds the brain to the energy needs and status of our 20 trillion cells. Leptin resistance also prevents control of how calories are partitioned to our peripheral cells. Leptin does something else is interesting. Leptin resistance alters the receptors that control the wiring and firing of our reward tracts in the brain. This is why obese people with leptin resistance tend to have abnormally low levels of dopamine receptors in the reward tracts, making them slaves to high-reward foods such as processed carbohydrates.

The other part of this story is the role of gut bacteria. In obesity, the composition of gut flora becomes simplified compared to optimal colonization from an ancestral diet. Today's western diets consist of heavily processed foods that are made from industrial polyunsaturated fats, processed proteins, and chemically modified starches, all of which are digested and absorbed before reaching the colon. In fact, most of our carbohydrates these days are digested and fully absorbed within the first two feet of our intestine. This is not how ancestral diets were digested. The ancestral diet included extensive roots and tubers that underwent tedious digestion well beyond the first two feet of our GI tract. Today's chemically simplified foods create an overly simplified gut flora.

Also, overly simplified gut flora leads to the production of more short-chain fatty acids (SCFA), instead of naturally selecting for stool-forming gut bacteria. This is why we have seen a huge spike in colon cancer in the United States since 1900. Normal colon bacteria turn SCFA into anti-inflammatory omega-3 fats. If you do not have those beneficial bacteria in your colon because your diet is processed, your omega-6 to omega-3 ratio rises, creating a cellular terrain for cancer. In 1900, colon cancer was the 37th leading cause of death in the United States. Today it is the second leading cause of death.

Also, because processed food is absorbed much faster, bypassing the normal gut hormone response, this allows it to evade the normal signaling pathways in the brain via leptin receptors. This ultimately leads to excessive weight gain, another reason the conventional notion of "a calorie is a calorie" is just not true.

In the heart, HS-CRP fosters the development of atheroma, or fatty deposits, in the coronary arteries and the stiffening of heart valves. Over time it also causes huge changes to the heart's electrical system, leading to arrhythmia generation. This is why atrial fibrillation is so common in America today. Eventually the atheroma collects oxidized LDL and grows until it causes a plaque to explode, causing a heart attack or death. The plaque is the dynamite, and the HS-CRP is the lit match. Neither one is dangerous unless they are present together.

Understanding how the brain-gut axis functions is a study in how our liver protects us. Our liver is the last line of defense before toxins assault the brain. Once the brain is impacted, hormonal disruption ensues, beginning with leptin resistance and cascading to every other hormone. The brain loses control over cellular homeostasis, and Neolithic diseases take root.

We can understand this process when we look out our VAP profiles in context of our diet and our light and time cycles. The VAP measurements don't really measure lipids in my view. It is a test that tells us how well our brain-gut axis is functioning to protect the 20 trillion cells in our body from disease propagation. This is how the Epi-paleo Rx uses it.

8. Homocysteine

Homocysteine always should be considered in cardiovascular, neurological, and osteological (bone) disease work ups. This test has become controversial, but I still think it is one of the better and cheaper tests for a biohack. Homocysteine is a metabolite of the amino acid methionine, a building block of cells. The breakdown of homocysteine cannot be completed if there is a lack of vitamins B6, folic acid, B12, and betaine. Correcting the appropriate deficiency that causes high homocysteine often relieves symptoms of fatigue, balance problems and sleep disturbance. High homocysteine is a reliable marker of inflammation, especially in the cases of osteoporosis and cardiovascular disease. Homocysteine also is elevated in those with stroke risk and neurodegenerative disorders. This is the inflammatory link that ties cardiovascular risk and diseases such as Alzheimer's and stroke together. I have found that when someone has leptin resistance, homocysteine is a very reliable indication of inflammation at a cellular level.

Homocysteine is currently under scientific attack. The most recent Cochrane Review concluded there is no evidence that reducing homocysteine with B vitamins alone will reduce cardiovascular risk. I believe this is accurate, but I like to use homocysteine levels as a proxy for what is going on at an epigenetic level. When it is elevated it is usually a sign that we are turning on or off genes via a process called methylation. Low levels of inflammation do not support high homocysteine, so when we can't rely on HS-CRP or ferritin, we can use homocysteine as a failsafe in our biohack.

I still test mine to for insight on what might be going on at my DNA level because of all the damage I inflicted on my body in my former lifestyle.

Another reason I check homocysteine is because of the increased dietary folic acid levels in this country due to enriched grains. The more folic acid we eat, the higher our risk is of developing a high homocysteine level. This has become a huge issue nationally since grain manufacturers began adding folic acid to grains in 1998 to lower spina bifida risks. Unfortunately, this has altered methylation processes and affected the epigenetic switch settings on our genes. This has increased our risks for several cancers by increasing inflammation.

9. Complete CBC with differential and platelet count (sometimes an Ivy bleeding time)

This is a straight-forward biohack. Here we are looking at our oxygen carrying capacity and seeing if there are reversible causes of anemia related to diet. The white count often times will give us insight to a possible gut infection or an infection somewhere else in the body. This is especially true if we see an abnormally low total cholesterol without statin use and a mild anemia. Many times iron deficiency anemia can be tied to excessive dairy use as well.

10. Gender-specific hormone panels, serum and salivary

For hormone panels I run cortisol, total testosterone, free testosterone, % free testosterone, Dihydrotestosterone (DHT), luteinizing hormone (LH), follicle-stimulating hormone (FSH), estradiol (E2), Dehydroepiandrosterone sulfate (DHEA-S), prostate-specific antigen (PSA), insulin-like growth factor (IGF-1), and, very rarely, a serum leptin level.

I consider them all based on levels of progesterone, pregnenolone, melatonin, serum and urine osmolarity, prolactin levels, and melanocyte-stimulating hormone (MSH). I usually decide what tests to order based on each clinical scenario. You can order any or every one of these and hand the results to your doctor for help. But you can also teach yourself what these mean. It's not that hard! Whether you doctor knows what to do with these tests is immaterial. They will need to get you to someone who can. That is their job. These labs are critical in deciphering where the inflammation is coming from to cause Neolithic disease. They are not used this way currently in medicine. This is an epic mistake in my view. I want to teach you why they are important so you know how to use this information to get the care you need and require.

What characterizes susceptibility to disease?

Hormones levels give you insight into the effects of food and your environment on your current biochemistry. I like to call this the Rosetta Stone of how to figure out what is really going on. We know clearly that we can alter our DNA switches by changing our diet. We can use exercise to do this, too, but nothing is more effective than dietary alteration. Food quality and choices dictate 95 percent of our genetic expression. Diet is that important!

Most physicians and patients believe disease risk is set by genetics. This is false, but also the most common excuse doctors give patients when we do not know the answer. We just blame it on genetics and hope you're satisfied. Don't be. We learned this from the studies by Nir Barzilai, MD on super centenarians at Albert Einstein Medical College. Studies on people over 100 years old showed they were all found to harbor most of the bad genes we already know about. What was very interesting, however, was that the bad genes were turned off in these people. The ultimate arbiter of a long healthy life is the expression of our genes-whether they are turned on or off. This is called the epigenetic expression of disease.

11. Complete thyroid panel with antibody screening (TPO Ab and Tg Ab)

This is critical for the Hashimoto's hypothyroid patients, who make up the bulk of this disease hack.

A. TSH level, Free T4 and Free T3 ("free" means unbound fraction of hormone and is bio-available)

B. Reverse T3: To be done at the same time you do the Free T3. Then calculate your ratio with the results and measurements. Realize that most labs do not make these two the same units, so you will to find a calculator online to make that conversion.

C. Thyroid antibodies (TPO Ab and TgAb)

D. Four iron labs, which include Ferritin, % Saturation, TIBC and serum iron mentioned above.

12. Complete Urinalysis (beta HCG for menstruating women)

This includes a standard urinalysis, a urine specific gravity and regular chemistries.

13. Highly Sensitive CRP (HS-CRP)-not a regular CRP

This is well covered in the VAP section in this chapter.

14. Omega 6:3 serum test (for severe findings consider tissue assay)

This assay is critical before you change your diet and lifestyle to see how far you need to go with the Paleolithic diet. It generally takes 12-36 months to reverse this ratio depending upon how gone you are. When I began I was at 35:1 and it took me three years to get below a 4:1 ratio.

15. Fasting serum insulin and HbA1c assessment

I generally do this as a baseline test and order it frequently if I have a diabetic who wants to reverse his or her disease.

16. Complete Vitamin D3 panel-vitamin D3, the immunity steroid

In a Epi-paleo Rx biohack, levels of vitamin D3, or cholecalciferol, are used to evaluate the immune system and the synthesis of hormones from LDL cholesterol. Vitamin D is the last hormone in the chain of steroid hormones, so if it is not in the optimal range, it tells me something is wrong somewhere in the system. It is a very important part of the Epi-paleo Rx to understand how important Vitamin D is in our systems, so we are going to go into some detail.

Low vitamin D levels signal that I need to find out why they are low. You must get this lab with an HS-CRP. I call HS-CRP the "fire indicator" for inflammation. Vitamin D is the "water" that puts out the fire. Ideally, we would like our vitamin D level in the optimal range of 60-100 ng/ml and HS-CRP as close to zero as possible. Any variation in those variables means we have work to do.

One of vitamin D's most important actions is to modulate the immune system, as receptors for vitamin D are found on T helper cells. These are the same cells that HIV wipes out in AIDS victims. A vitamin D deficiency turns off the epigenetic switches that protect us from viruses, bacteria, and fungal infections. In fact, since I got my level checked five years ago, I have not been seriously ill since.

Diseases associated with low vitamin D levels-below 30 ng/ml on a 25-hydroxyvitamin D test:

- Rickets, osteomalacia, and psoriasis
- Hypocalcemia
- Seizures, muscle tetanus, and heart failure in the newly born
- Osteoporosis and osteopenia
- Cancer of all types
- Heart disease (the number-one killer of men and women)
- High blood pressure
- Obesity
- Osteo/Rheumatoid Arthritis
- Mental illness of all types
- Chronic pain
- Muscular weakness
- Radiation poisoning
- Diabetes, especially metabolic syndrome and type 2 diabetes
- Multiple sclerosis and most autoimmune diseases

WHAT DOES VITAMIN D REALLY DO?

1. Vitamin D facilitates increased intestinal absorption of phosphorus and calcium as well as suppression of parathyroid hormone (PTH) secretion to increase our plasma calcium concentrations. It does not, however, dictate where this calcium will deposit in our bodies.

2. Vitamin D levels above 50 ng/ml are associated with increased adiponectin levels. High adiponectin means you are less likely to be obese. It also means your leptin levels are low. So higher vitamin D levels can help us trim our fat stores. Decreasing fat can help us avoid insulin resistance and the eventual development of type 2 diabetes.

3. It is a natural antibiotic that helps white blood cells clear infections. It does this by stimulating immune cells to make a protein called cathelicidin, which is found on T cells, macrophages, neutrophils, and on epithelial cells in our guts and respiratory system. It helps defend us from viruses and bacteria. In the gut lining it activates T regulator cells to protect the intestinal lining and the GALT that lies behind the brush border. It now appears that low vitamin D in the gut may be a risk factor for developing

an HIV infection. Vitamin D also blocks the intracellular inflammatory signals of NF Kappa beta and of TNF alpha, both of which play a role in many pathologic diseases, such as cancer, autoimmunity, and obesity.

4. Vitamin D inhibits the hormone renin in our kidneys, which helps prevent high blood pressure. It also protects the kidney from high levels of uric acid production that come from end-stage fructose metabolism.

5. Usually the skin makes 10,000-20,000 IU of vitamin D. Excess Vitamin D 3 is then broken down to its degradation products. These degradation products have been shown to inhibit psoriasis by preventing the skin from reproducing at a faster rate than normal, the pathology found in psoriasis. The lower epidermis grows 25-40 times faster, creating a large red plaque on the surface. This is why light therapy is so effective in treating psoriasis. Anyone with psoriasis should check their Vitamin D levels before doing anything else, as most have extremely low levels, tend to be obese, and have higher cancer rates, as well.

6. In autoimmune diseases we need to advocate for much higher levels of Vitamin D. Why? In order for circulating vitamin D to perform its functions, it must first activate the vitamin D receptor (VDR). The problem is that many people with autoimmune disease have a genetic polymorphism that affects the expression and activation of the VDR, thus reducing the biologic activity of vitamin D. Studies have shown that a significant number of patients with autoimmune diseases have several VDR polymorphisms. If you have a VDR problem you require much higher circulating levels of vitamin D to bind to these defective receptors. As I have mentioned in multiple blogs, a leaky gut predisposes one to the development of autoimmunity. Moreover, optimal vitamin D levels are also linked to tighter junctions in the intestinal lining, making our guts less leaky. If the gut is less leaky, the immune system is stronger because it does not have to be activated constantly to protect the rest of the body. Vitamin D also plays a huge role in the immune surveillance of our GI tracts. It appears to be critical to push your levels to a much higher plasma level with VDR problem. The fears of toxicity are overblown in my estimation, and the risks associated with low vitamin D are far too common.

There is recent evidence from Hector DeLuca, PhD, DSc, MD about multiple sclerosis and autoimmune encephalitis, an autoimmune disease in which the immune system attacks brain tissue. DeLuca believes the degradation products of vitamin D and some byproducts of solar radiation are active against a range of autoimmune illnesses, including multiple sclerosis. I have always felt that MS, ALS and Guillian-Barre are tied in to vitamin D metabolism. It appears DeLuca believes this, as well. I think Wahls' insight into her cure is a critical piece that we must add to the clinical quilt of treating autoimmune disease.

7. Vitamin D is a fat-soluble molecule. Make sure your vitamin D is not packaged in an omega-6 oil as most are. Since it is fat-soluble, you should take it with fat for absorption. But it also means that some people will not absorb it well. Who? Those with a leaky gut, inflammatory bowel disease, Crohn's, ulcerative colitis, liver disease, no gallbladder, those on a low-fat diet, and those on NSAIDs, steroids longer than a two weeks, blood thinners, anticoagulants, reflux medicines and antacids, and synthetic hormones such as birth control pills. Do you see why we have an epidemic of low vitamin D now?

8. Can you have a normal plasma D level and still have low vitamin D activity? Yes, and it is probably the biggest silent epidemic today. I most commonly see this in obese people with hypothyroidism. Ninety percent of the cases of hypothyroidism in the United States are cause by Hashimoto's disease, an autoimmune disease. These patients universally have defective VDR receptors. That means they need very high levels of blood Vitamin D levels and optimization of thyroid function for results. Many obese people get stuck not losing weight because their doctors think their thyroid and vitamin D levels are fine when their levels are sub-therapeutic. Many patients find amazing results when their plasma levels are pushed higher. I also see this in post-op cancer patients under extreme stress, and patients with high cortisol levels.

9. Age will decrease your skin's ability to make vitamin D from sunlight and cholesterol. As we go from age 20 to 60 we lose that ability by a four-fold magnitude. The darker our skin the worse the conversion is. So as we age, we need more sun or supplementation, not less of either. This is why so many older people see a higher incidence of Neolithic disease.

10. Humans have a vitamin D savings bank in the body. A good protein diet leads to a better vitamin D level and a Paleolithic diet is an optimal choice for this bank account. It works by making a protein called vitamin D binding protein (DBP), a highly specific carrier for vitamin D and all of its metabolites found in the plasma. This allows us to store vast amounts of vitamin D. If we are protein deficient we do not have this ability and our

stores are low in low-light levels. It not only protects our vitamin D stores, but it also prevents the toxic effects of a high vitamin D level in the blood. Humans store vitamin D when levels are above 40 ng/ml. The interesting finding is that it is only around a level of 60 ng/ml that the stores are sufficient to see us through a winter at an optimal D level. This is why dietary composition is critical for immunity, and why flu season peaks in winter months. Those with low HDL levels or liver disease tend to make the lowest amounts of DBP, such as in patients with hepatitis or metabolic syndrome.

11. Higher vitamin D levels are associated with longer telomere lengths. This means that optimal vitamin D levels reduce cellular aging, reduce the use of our stem cells, and decrease the leakiness of our mitochondria. If your vitamin D level is low your telomeres will be shortened, putting you at heightened risk for faster aging and Neolithic disease.

12. When you optimize your vitamin D you will notice your HDL level will rise 10-30 percent in the first year. This signifies the liver is doing a better job of "skimming" the portal circulation for endotoxins. This is the major mechanism for Vitamin D's protection of the heart in my view. We hear doctors say a high HDL protects the heart. This is how-by making the liver a master of defense. It also protects the brain from endotoxin assault and is a main defense in the brain-gut axis. Read my VAP blog to freshen up on this physiology.

13. I have just skimmed the surface here why vitamin D does a ton more than I learned in medical school 20 years ago. I keep reading about it because we are learning new things daily. Consider this: the ApoE4 allele is the allele that gave humans the ability to leave Africa and live in lower levels of solar radiation yet still capture enough Vitamin D to survive. This allele is associated with other diseases but it was ideally matched for humans who needed to migrate north and south from the equator.

It is also vitally important for our immunity and defense. Studies show vitamin D decreased the risk of breast cancer in women when their levels were over 50 ng/ml. This has huge implications for all women and all oncologists in my view. It also improves athletic performance. The 2010 Chicago Blackhawks became the first team to have their Vitamin D levels maintained all season long via diet and supplementation and they won the Stanley Cup. They also had the fewest injuries and games missed due to illness in the entire league by a large margin. They changed their protocol because one of the players' wives saw a physician who knew how vitamin

D enhances athletic performance. The news spread to many other major professional franchises and several implemented changes to their offseason regimens. Two of those teams were the NFL's Green Bay Packers and the Pittsburg Steelers. By the way, both optimized their Vitamin D status and both played in the Super bowl the same year (Feb 2011). Coincidence? Maybe it is. But I will let you decide how to use this information.

IN CONCLUSION

You also need a thorough history and physical exam, and to retest on a quarterly or biannual basis. This will provide feedback on your regimen so you can adjust and get things right over time. How often you do these things should be based upon your results. If you are meeting with no success you need to look for new problems.

Once this is all correlated, you then come up with a customized dietary plan, sometimes calling for medications or supplements, and an exercise plan that fits your current cardiovascular fitness profile. You basically make a game plan for things to alter for optimal health. It should be a collaboration between you and your doctor or other health care provider.

This is a very labor-intensive task for both patient and doctor. But if you remain persistent and consistent, always focusing on your health, you can reach any goal you set. It must be adaptable yet have the core values that will get you to The Promised Land. The secret sauce is not the lab list; it is found in the interpretation of those labs and how they correlate with your epigenetic switches. That is what determines how your body partitions calories and which diet and exercise program are best for your current biology. You should expect this to change over time as you become optimized. Nothing stays they same in biology. I learned this on my own journey and it has proven true in those I have helped re-engineer themselves back to optimal. Enjoy!

REFERENCES

1. G. Toperoff, D. Aran, J. D. Kark, M. Rosenberg, T. Dubnikov, B. Nissan, J. Wainstein, Y. Friedlander, E. Levy-Lahad, B. Glaser, A. Hellman. Genome-wide survey reveals predisposing diabetes type 2-related DNA methylation variations in human peripheral blood. Human Molecular Genetics, 2011; 21 (2): 371 DOI: 10.1093/hmg/ddr472

2. Berg RD. The indigenous gastrointestinal microflora. Trends Microbiol1996;4:430-5.

3. Hultberg M. Cysteine turnover in human cell lines is influenced by glyphosate (2007) Environmental Toxicology and Pharmacology, 24 (1), pp. 19-22.

4. http://www.cps.ca/english/statements/ii/fnim07-01.htm

5. Godel JC, Hart AG. Northern infant syndrome: A deficiency state? Can Med Assoc J 1984;131:199-204.

6. Haworth JC, Dilling LA. Vitamin-D-deficient rickets in Manitoba, 1972-84. CMAJ 1986;134:237-41.

7. Lebrun JB, Moffatt ME, Mundy RJ, et al. Vitamin D deficiency in a Manitoba community. Can J Public Health 1993;84:394-6.

8. Ward LM, Gaboury I, Ladhani M, Zlotkin S. Vitamin D-deficiency rickets among children in Canada. CMAJ 2007;177:161-6.

9. Weiler HA, Leslie WD, Krahn J, Steiman PW, Metge CJ. Canadian Aboriginal women have a higher prevalence of vitamin D deficiency than non-Aboriginal women despite similar dietary vitamin D intakes. J Nutr 2007;137:461-5.

10. Canadian Paediatric Society, First Nations and Inuit Health Committee [Principal author: J Godel]. Vitamin D supplementation in northern Native communities. Paediatr Child Health 2002;7:459-63.

11. Holick MF. Vitamin D: Its role in cancer prevention and treatment. Prog Biophys Mol Biol 2006;92:49-59.

12. Zittermann A. Vitamin D in preventive medicine: Are we ignoring the evidence? Br J Nutr 2003;89:552-72.

13. Javaid MK, Crozier SR, Harvey NC, et al; Princess Anne Hospital Study Group. Maternal vitamin D status during pregnancy and childhood bone mass at age 9 years: A longitudinal study. Lancet 2006;367:36-43. (Erratum in 2006;367:1486).

14. Camargo CA Jr, Rifas-Shiman SL, Litonjua AA, et al. Maternal intake of vitamin D during pregnancy and risk of recurrent wheeze at 3 y of age. Am J Clin Nutr 2007;85:788-95.

15. Munger KL, Zhang SM, O'Reilly E, et al. Vitamin D intake and incidence of multiple sclerosis. Neurology 2004;62:60-5.

16. Sinnott BP, Licata AA. Assessment of bone and mineral metabolism in inflammatory bowel disease: Case series and review. Endocr Pract 2006;12:622-9.

Chapter Six

DISEASE ONE: OSTEOPOROSIS / OSTEOPENIA

BAD TO THE BONE

In my day job as a neurosurgeon, I operate on a lot of diseased spines. In the last 12 years I have repaired more than 1,000 vertebral column fractures from osteoporosis or osteopenia. In May of 2011, I did a podcast interview with blogger Jimmy Moore about the link between diet, bone metabolism, and Neolithic disease. I talked about the dramatic increases in the incidences of osteoporosis I had seen, which drove me to look for the underlying cause.

Many people think since bones are hard they are not an active tissue in our body. This is not true. Bone is a very active tissue that constantly turns over. We continually lay down new bone in response to stressors and resorb bone from areas that are not stressed. Since bone is so active, it uses massive amounts of energy. This is where leptin comes in. Any tissue that requires a ton of energy is coupled to leptin biochemistry. The story on bones and osteoporosis, however, is a very complicated one. This osteoporosis chapter will have many twists and turns. Most spine surgeons won't know much of what you are going to learn here because the interconnectedness of the body's systems are not taught in medical school. Most physicians do not link osteoporosis with leptin resistance-just ask one and see.

CONVENTIONAL WISDOM FOR OSTEOPOROSIS

Most doctors will tell you to take calcium and vitamin D and to exercise to treat osteoporosis. They may prescribe a bisphosphonate drug, too, such as Fosamax, Actonel, Boniva, and Aredia. I don't use these drugs at all. If you take them you can bet you won't cure a thing and you may even make the problem worse. These drugs have a large side effect profile and are linked with some pretty steep complications, such as bone cancer in the jaw, fractures of the femur bone, and esophageal cancers. Most physicians are taught that osteoporosis is a geriatric disease seen most often in postmenopausal women or in men with obstructive lung disease. Most know that hormone deficits play a role in this condition, but few treat their patients for this deficiency because of several flawed studies that have made my profession skittish about hormone replacement therapy. They may know that smoking increases the risk of developing the disease, as well. Doctors will place you on 1,000-1,400 mg of calcium daily, 50,000 IU of Vitamin D2, and perhaps a magnesium supplement. They also may order a DEXA bone scan to assess your risk. That is about where the current conventional treatment ends.

WHAT DOES OSTEOPOROSIS LOOK LIKE THROUGH A EPI-PALEO RX PRISM?

For many years I never appreciated how a gut issue could cause osteoporosis in young people. When we encountered it in training, it was usually blamed on genetics, old age, or menopause. My thoughts changed about seven years ago when a woman under the age 30 of came into the emergency room with severe osteoporosis. She was partially paralyzed due to advanced degenerative disc disease and a broken vertebrae in her neck, despite no trauma. Her case revolutionized my perspective as she had none of the classic risk factors. I wanted to know why it happened to her.

By that point in my career, I viewed things differently and was open to other causes of her disease. I discovered her bone condition was related to her diet of processed foods from the fast-food restaurants she frequented. She had extremely low vitamin D levels, an elevated HS-CRP, very low testosterone, and very high estrogen levels. She also had terrible sleep issues and her cortisol pattern was completely backwards compared to normal labs. She also had a terrible body composition, even though she was at a good weight for her height.

I had to take her to surgery immediately and stabilize her neck with an operation. During surgery, I found her bone was very poor quality. The first thing we did post-operatively was put her on a Paleolithic diet high in animal protein and medium chain triglyceride (MCT) fat. We also added vitamins D3 and K2 to her medication list. We added some minerals because she could not absorb them from food due to her leaky gut. She magically improved in just over 18 months, and really helped me change the way I looked at all spinal disorders as a neurosurgeon. I think I learned more from her case than any case in my training. It taught me to look at the origin of disease, since she fit none of the established criteria. That case haunted me.

THE UNCONVENTIONAL CAUSE IN HER CASE: SAD

Primary care physicians and spine surgeons are taught a law called Wolff's law of bone formation. It says the more stressed a bone is, the more bone is laid down, and the stronger the bone is. This law is why most spine surgeons don't expect obese patients will have osteoporosis, yet these are the people experiencing a silent epidemic of this Neolithic disease. The numbers of people with osteoporosis exploded during the last 30 years. I think I had a one-hour lecture on osteoporosis in medical school, and now it is involved in close to 80 percent of my cases. Few spine surgeons expect to see osteoporosis in younger patients because they think it is a disease in older women with low estrogen. Nevertheless, we often see it on MRIs as loss of mineral content and more fat in the marrow space of long bones and spinal bones. Spine surgeons must be more vigilant about this disease and its links to the leptin hormone.

Here are some random dietary facts about osteoporosis in humans:

When your diet has a lot of:

- Total protein, you have a 3.6 times lower risk of fracture. Protein seems to be a potential Primal Rx cure, but lets look further.
- Animal protein, you have a 4.5 times lower risk of fracture, so eating grass fed meat is critical.
- Vegetable protein, you have you have a 2.9 times INCREASED risk of fracture, so vegetable protein does not equal animal protein!
- Carbohydrates, you have a 4.9 times INCREASED risk of fractures. Nothing increase your risk for fracture more than excessive carbs!

These basic facts point out why what you eat can put you at risk for your bones disappearing, no matter your age or sex. Fats also play a huge role. Good fats are the basis of cholesterol that can be converted to the hormones your bones need for strength. These hormones are DHEA, testosterone, estrogen, and progesterone. Optimizing these hormones is part of the Primal Rx, as you will see shortly.

Diet affects the two main cells that are involved in bone metabolism, osteoblasts and osteoclasts. Osteoblasts lay bone down and osteoclasts resorb bone. Osteoporosis can be caused by poor bone apposition (laying bone down), by resorption (breaking down) of the bone, or a combination of both. Most of the bisphosphonate drugs work on osteoclasts to stop them from resorbing the bone. There are only two synthetic drugs that use anabolic (bone-building) mechanisms to make new bone. One is a human-cloned hormone called parathyroid hormone (PTH), and the other is the drug Forteo. Forteo is a synthetic drug with many risks and side effects. I do use it in high-risk cases, but not often.

Bone cells are controlled by the hormones leptin, testosterone, estrogen, progesterone, and cortisol, but there are many more major players as you will soon find out. Progesterone is particularly effective in stopping bone resorption in both men and postmenopausal women, although it seems many health care providers are not aware of this. Low progesterone is a bigger deal than low estrogen for postmenopausal women. I believe the reason this information is not used is because of the horribly flawed data from the Women's Health Initiative study that came out in 2002. A study of hormone replacement therapy that was flawed in many ways, it has done more to set back the optimal treatment of osteoporosis in older populations than any other study. You need to be aware of this situation.

Because diet is critical to osteoporosis, we should start this journey in the gastrointestinal tract. In October 2011, Gastroeneterology published a paper that gave more credence to my thoughts on how osteoporosis should be treated today. This paper shows that food absorption in the GI tract directly influences bone mass. That evidence came from the study of ATF4, a transcription factor found in osteoblasts, the bone-forming cells. ATF4 is required for osteoblasts to function and make new bone. It affects bone formation, including extracellular matrix synthesis, osteoclast differentiation, and the energy metabolism that is overseen by leptin function. ATF4 also is needed for amino acid import into cells, which are the building blocks in protein and what bone is made from.

Experiments in mice and humans have shown that diets high animal protein and fat tend to overcome low ATF4 levels in the gut. High-fat diets are also bone healthy because fats are required to make the hormones that protect the bones; sex steroid hormones and vitamin D all are derived from LDL cholesterol. This is another major reason I'm completely against the use of statins in humans. Many people with osteoporosis are also on statins, and I think this is a problem. If you have this disease you might want to consider talking to you physician to stop statins and start on fish oil and niacin instead. This is a good replacement for a statin if your physician is adamant you take it.

The most important dietary risk for osteoporosis appears to be a high-carbohydrate, low-fat, and low-protein diet, which causes osteoporosis all by itself! Ironically, this is the diet outlined in the USDA pyramid or plate, designed by Walter Willet, a famous Harvard-based nutritionist. It is also the diet Dean Ornish and most vegans advocate. Willet is considered an expert on diet, but his work, in my opinion, has caused more Neolithic disease than one could imagine. The effects of the standard American diet (SAD) explains my clinical findings during the last 15 years in my spine practice. I found that people with altered body compositions are found during surgery or on MRIs to have bad bone health. This was not what I was taught to expect in medical school or during my spine training. I was taught that a stressed bone placed under a load should be made stronger over time, and that fat people should have great bones. Yet within one year of practice I was overwhelmed by patients of all ages and body types who had osteoporosis. I since learned that if one is leptin resistant, Wolff's law is null and void. This is the number-one rule of my Primal osteoporosis Rx and everything flows from this rule. Many physicians do not realize this, which is why this disease goes untreated so long and has become a national epidemic. If you do not know to look for it, it is hard to diagnose.

LITTLE-KNOWN HORMONES INVOLVED IN BONE HEALTH

Recently, Gerard Karsenty, MD, PhD, and his colleagues at Columbia University Medical Center discovered osteoblasts (bone-forming cells) secrete a hormone called osteocalcin, which regulates insulin production and enhances insulin sensitivity to protect our bones. It also increases testosterone, which increases bone density in both men and women.

Osteocalcin is vital in forming bone and directing calcium deposition in bone, dentin (teeth), and the arteries of our body. There is even scientific evidence of a hypothalamic pituitary axis that controls our susceptibility to tooth decay and dental plaque and the mineralization of teeth. This was work done 25 years ago by Dr. John Lenora of Loma Linda University.

Osteocalcin is also tied to a vitamin found in food called vitamin K2. Vitamin K2 is not like the vitamin K1 with which most physicians are familiar. In fact, many do not know that vitamin K has three isoforms, and all three do different things. Vitamin K2 has been removed from the modern food supply by food processing. Vitamin K2 and osteocalcin are key factors in saliva to help maintain optimal dental health.

In essence, osteocalcin sends absorbed calcium to the correct tissues in our body. This is important because the conventional wisdom treatment for osteoporosis usually involves only calcium and vitamin D supplementation. Recent studies have linked calcium supplementation to adverse cardiac outcomes. The reason for this link is not well known, but it is likely secondary to a co-morbid lack of vitamin K2 in people, perhaps causing calcium to be sent to our coronary and carotid arteries instead of our bone. Vitamin K2 is the calcium traffic cop in our bodies, and osteocalcin tells us whether we are deficient in this vitamin. You can order this test yourself off the internet without a prescription and bring it to your doctor's attention.

In order to become active, osteocalcin has to be carboxylated, a chemical reaction that adds carbon dioxide or bicarbonate to form a carboxyl group. When someone has insulin resistance or type 2 diabetes, they have a lot of un-carboxylated osteocalcin, which won't allow calcium into the bone collagen matrix. This is another reason diabetics are at high risk for bone diseases. Instead, the calcium is placed in tissues where it doesn't belong, such as heart valves and in many different arteries of our body. Most aortic valves in this country are replaced because they are calcified and don't work. Why? They are vitamin K2 deficient. This link is not well known by vascular surgeons. I have alerted my colleagues about this link so they can help patients who have arterial calcification. I often see this risk when I see X-rays that show calcification of arteries. Most people with bad atherosclerosis also suffer from this. This can be followed up and measured with a calcium index score of your heart or vessels-a high calcium index score is not a good sign for your long-term health. This is particularly true for your heart.

We want this calcium to be directed to our bone and not the soft tissues in our vascular tree. This is why studies have found excessive calcium supplementation to be harmful. The answer is to stop the calcium supplementation and take K2 through diet or supplementation. Most people who have had their gallbladders removed also have a vitamin K2 deficiency because the body recycles K2 using the gallbladder. I have an entire blog on my website that covers the K2 recycle steps if you would like to learn more about how this might effect your health.

So what carboxylates osteocalcin to make it active in humans? Vitamin K2! K2 carboxylates osteocalcin to make it an active hormone to direct calcium to the right tissues. When K2 levels are low, we see calcification in the arteries, the spine, or as tartar build up on your teeth. This is information few physicians and dentists are aware of. I learned about it in piecemeal fashion because I was a dentist before I was a neurosurgeon, and I put those pieces together about seven years ago. My teeth used to build up a lot of tartar until I increased my K2 levels in my diet and in supplement forms.

People with diabetes and insulin resistance are deficient in vitamin K2, as are most people who eat a SAD. Because osteocalcin helps modulate insulin release, vitamin K2 can also be used to treat type 2 diabetes; there are several published studies on this, although they are also not well known in this country. The Japanese use vitamin K2 in the form of natto to treat osteoporosis.

I first discovered the link between K2 and osteoporosis while doing research related to my young patient with the broken neck I mentioned earlier. While looking for answers I tripped over this data. Like most physicians, I did not know what K2 was at that time, much less what it did. If you go into most pharmacies or supplement stores you will be hard pressed to find vitamin K2 even today. Allopathic medicine recognizes vitamin D3 deficiency, but in my opinion vitamin K2 deficiency is a bigger and more costly public health mess because it is common in three epidemic diseases: Diabetes, atherosclerosis, and osteoporosis. The cost of treating these diseases in our country is staggering. This is clearly an area where an ounce of prevention saves a pound of cures.

I use K2 frequently in my practice because most who come to see me have a spine disease. Vitamin K2 is on my top-ten Paleo supplement list on my blog. Most vascular surgeons are unaware of what vitamin K2 is and how it can prevent atherosclerosis. I run a lab on osteocalcin to quantify how much a patient's diet is depleted in vitamin K2. Most of our endogenous (made in the body) vitamin K1 and K2 is made from gut bacteria when we are healthy. But if you have a leaky gut or gut dysbiosis, you might not be able to recapture your vitamin K2 and will need a bigger dietary source on a regular basis. I think the SAD selects for a gut microflora that ensures vitamin K2 depletion, and that this is the reason we have a pandemic in vitamin K2 losses and see a lot of unhealthy bone. I also think it is why cardiovascular disease is so prevalent these days. Going with a Paleolithic diet solves this issue for most.

So if one has leptin resistance, leaky gut, or dysbiosis, we should expect a major problem with osteocalcin and K2 if we follow our own labs. I always look at the patient's HDL level to see if the gut may be leaky. I covered this extensively on the chapter on lab tests. Here is another thing to remember about Vitamin K-if the patient is on Coumadin, the problem is a bigger deal. Coumadin is a very common prescription and blocks the body's ability to recycle vitamin K, making it a very potent blood thinner, but also depleting cells of K2.

Vitamin K2 is important not only for diabetics, patients with heart disease, and patients with peripheral artery disease from atherosclerosis, but also for those with osteopenia or osteoporosis. Vitamin K2 is used as a first-line treatment of osteoporosis in Japan in doses of up to 45 mg a day. Unlike the SAD, the Japanese diet has a major source of Vitamin K2 in natto, which is fermented soybeans. Yes, I have tried it, and it tastes terrible. None of my patients will eat natto! The best source of Vitamin K2 in the SAD is pastured butter, which, ironically, most physicians advise their patients not to eat. Pastured butter is grass-fed butter. Vitamin K2 is also found in many green leafy plants, but with newer farming techniques and the advent of many pesticides, vitamin K levels have dropped in most non-organic foods.

Gut dysbiosis and leaky gut are the major causes of osteocalcin problems because K2 also comes from gut bacteria. If the gut flora mix is not optimal, we lose our ability to recycle endogenous vitamin K. This creates an overall depletion of Vitamin K that must be compensated for in our diet. In the United States, our diets have been stripped of vitamin K2, partly because pasteurization robs dairy products of their vitamin K content.

Raw dairy, on the other hand, contains plenty of vitamin K2. This is why I tell my osteopenic patients to seek raw milk and raw milk cheeses.

If we can't recycle our vitamin K2 and we have poor dietary sources of K2, it means the proteins that depend on K2 are not going to work optimally. We see the effects in the heart, arteries, and in our bones. So people who are deficient in K2 cannot activate osteocalcin. Moreover, the data from the experiments at Columbia University made it clear that osteocalcin tells our pancreatic beta cells to produce more insulin and our pituitary gland to make more testosterone. These two mechanisms help us form bone. This is exactly why the Primal Rx employs these techniques for treatment.

WHY POSTMENOPAUSAL WOMEN STRUGGLE WITH FAT LOSS

Osteocalcin has another little-known function important for diabetics and the obese. Osteocalcin instructs fat cells to release adiponectin, a hormone that increases our insulin sensitivity. Adiponectin is inversely correlated with body weight. It is highest in thin patients and lowest in the obese. This hormone plays a role in the metabolic derangements that result in type 2 diabetes, obesity, atherosclerosis, and fatty liver disease. Women also have higher levels of adiponectin than men, as well as higher levels of leptin. When adiponectin is released from fat cells, so is leptin.

These facts are important when one considers weight loss patterns in men and women and why they differ, and why women struggle with their weight after menopause. Another factor is declining dopamine levels, which control the release of hormones from the pituitary gland. This in turn affects the levels of dopamine in the reward tracts of the frontal lobes, causing people to seek foods that make them gain weight.

WHERE DOES LEPTIN FIT INTO THE OSTEOPOROSIS STORY?

Leptin is a hormone secreted by fat cells, and leptin inactivates osteocalcin via the sympathetic nervous system. Fat cells also release leptin when inflammation is high. Here is where I made the link between leptin resistance and osteoporosis about seven years ago. Leptin is very similar in chemical structure to IL-6, which is the main inflammatory cytokine behind many Neolithic diseases. This is the chemical that causes a person's hormone pattern to become altered on lab tests. When I realized this, I realized I could translate what was going on in the cells if I followed their hormone responses over time. I call this my Rosetta Stone moment!

High leptin sets the stage for insulin resistance to develop. Once insulin resistance is firmly entrenched, our liver loses control of a key enzyme called phosphoenolpyruvate carboxykinase (PEPCK). As a result, it begins to make excess triglycerides and HS-CRP, and release excessive ferritin. That is why I follow all these labs when I am bio-hacking a person. Now you can, too!

PEPCK is the master controller of gluconeogenesis, or the synthesis of glucose, in our liver. Most Neolithic diseases involve the loss of control of this enzyme when there is an alteration between energy generation, intracellular magnesium levels, and ATP. After several years of insulin resistance, other inflammatory cytokines such as TNF alpha, TNF beta, and IL-6 cause our adrenal glands to malfunction. This is called adrenal resistance, and means our cortisol levels have become altered from their normal pattern. You can check this best with a salivary cortisol level, not a serum or blood level. Cortisol should be highest in the morning and then gradually decline to be lowest at night. Very few MDs know this information, although neurosurgeons are familiar with assessing cortisol because we treat Cushing's syndrome, a disease in which pituitary tumors secrete cortisol. Harvey Cushing is considered the father of American neurosurgery.

Chronic leptin resistance drives daily cortisol levels ever higher, which stimulates the production of even more inflammatory cytokines. The process begins to feed upon itself. This is why diabetes is so hard to eradicate, but easy to treat with medicines like metformin or insulin. If you want to stay diabetic, you should follow the conventional advice of taking your medications. If you want to cure the disease, you need to immediately change to a ketogenic version of the Paleolithic diet. This is how I cured two of my own family members of this disease. They no longer take any diabetic medications.

As this process speeds along, leptin resistance develops all over the body. It occurs in the brain, liver, and in the muscle, radically affecting your metabolism. By this time, a doctor likely has diagnosed you with type 2 diabetes and wants you to take medications and follow the American

Diabetes Association diet. If you do this you will become a medica
and have zero chance of curing your disease.

Cortisol is one of the major hormones involved in the sympathe nervous system. The sympathetic nervous system is activated in acute and chronic stress response. Leptin resistance increases the sympathetic outflow from our brain. We are only designed to handle stress in smaller acute bursts, not on a chronic basis. When cortisol is secreted chronically at high levels in the face of multiple inflammatory cytokines, it's usually bad news. For example, you can develop early-onset menopause, andropause, sleep apnea, polycystic ovarian syndrome (PCOS), or adrenal fatigue (most MDs think this is woo-woo). Or you can go into a total system failure, such as fibromyalgia (many don't buy this diagnosis either). If you check any person with these diseases, one common lab pattern we see is low vitamin D, elevated HS-CRP, and very low DHEA levels. Now you know what to look for!

Very few physicians do this work up because they don't understand how cytokines affect hormones. Seven years ago I also had no clue how it all worked in unison. As a neurosurgeon, I only knew about the individual parts. However, this is the Rosetta Stone of the Primal Rx and it is critical you understand it.

HOW DOES THE ROSETTA STONE TRANSLATION WORK? SLEEP APNEA AS AN EXAMPLE

Low DHEA correlates with very high IL-6. There is a 98 percent correlation between IL-6 levels and decreased DHEA. This problem is best seen in those with sleep apnea who have ridiculously low DHEA levels, as low DHEA correlates with poor sleep. Poor sleep means you can't recycle old cellular parts, which is why people with sleep apnea die early, usually from cardiac disease. Each of the diseases mentioned above is associated with inflammatory cytokines that drive a hormonal imbalance. You fix that, you fix you. It's not hard. The best way to do it is to eat a primal diet. This is why the Primal Rx uses the Paleolithic diet as its core treatment. This is the only diet designed to run our Ferrari properly. If you gain nothing else in this book about all the biochemistry and endocrinology, but follow a strict Paleo diet, you will be better for it sooner or later depending upon how far from optimal you are. The key issue is the more inflammation you have in your cells the more hormonal abnormalities you have to overcome. Leptin

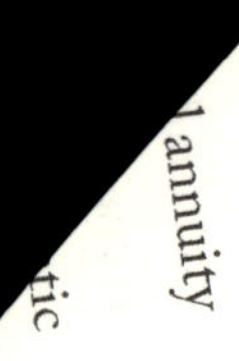

ı all back in order, but it may take five to seven years. the system works, you can use this book to help you . That is the Primal Rx promise.

THE BONE

When someone has chronic leptin resistance, they cannot carboxylate osteocalcin with K2. This blocks osteocalcin's main function to increase insulin production in the pancreas and increase testosterone production in the pituitary, which causes osteoporosis! This is one major reason obese people lose their bone quality and density. It also proves that Wolff's law is null and void when you are leptin resistant. The law remains true only when dealing with healthy conditions. In the United States, we have 60 million diabetics. Actually, I think the number is closer to 100 million, with 40 million insulin resistant people not yet formally diagnosed.

There is another cause of osteoporosis to add to this story-the chronic elevation of cortisol. When cortisol is chronically elevated together with insulin, you get deadly Neolithic diseases . The main reason is that chronic elevations of both hormones allow huge amounts of inflammation to enter the gut and pound the liver (our great protector), which is already spewing out tons of inflammatory byproducts. This is why the VAP cholesterol labs are so critical for you to understand how to hack yourself.

When the liver, our guardian that protects our circulation from free radical generation, is not functioning well, it causes our blood plasma to become oxidized. This creates the perfect situation for any Neolithic disease you can imagine. This process, I have found, is what causes so many of the spinal diseases I treat daily. I employ now what I know will cure them. It is possible for the person willing to follow the Primal Rx.

Now perhaps you understand why leptin is the kingpin hormone in this entire cascade. You can diagnose and figure out how best to cure any disease using this viewpoint. When I realized this, I transformed everything I did for my family and myself. It eventually transformed my practice of neurosurgery too. It can transform any disease you face today. I decided to write down all this knowledge of "connectiveness" in a document on my website called The Quilt. I did this to explain how all the individual pathways work together to either keep us healthy or allow us to develop Neolithic disease. In medicine and research circles, we learn about these parts by themselves, but do not learn how they work in unison. I realized all this after finding the real cause of osteoporosis in my practice. It wa that whatever controlled energy production in the body was the king That was leptin. Leptin sits at the top of my Quilt treatise for this reason

When I diagnose osteoporosis or osteopenia today, it is a sign to me multiple organ systems in the person are dying slowly, not just bone. Leptin, it turns out, is the "Ferrari brake" that prevents osteocalcin and insulin levels from becoming too high. People who are leptin resistant (obese) have high leptin levels, and this causes a rise in mitogen-activated protein kinase (JNK). JNKs do many things in our bodies. One major function is to respond to inflammatory cytokines such as IL-6. Chemically, leptin and IL-6 look very similar to one another. Also, in the GI tract JNK directly inhibits ATF4, effectively turning off all osteoblastic formation. So we cannot make more bone if we are leptin resistant, even if our diet is loaded with good foods. This was an astounding realization and completely explained what I had been seeing in my clinic for the last 15 years. It was my epiphany for this disease, my young patient, and my own problems!

Also, leptin resistance leads to high cortisol levels, which cause us to resorb bone faster than normal, worsening the osteopenia to osteoporosis. Most people know that excessive steroid use can cause osteoporosis, too. When steroids are given to people with leptin resistance and already high cortisol, we see the worst cases of osteoporosis you can imagine. Remember my 30-year-old patient at the beginning of this chapter? She was one of those patients. You are now a primal endocrinologist and bone specialist.

THE PRIMAL OSTEOPOROSIS RX

1. High cortisol must be brought back to normal. The most common reason for high cortisol today is leptin resistance from a SAD loaded with carbohydrates. Adopting a high-fat and high-protein Paleolithic diet is the first treatment option in most cases. Renal osteodystrohy is one of the few cases in which protein must be limited, but fats can be used liberally to support bone mass. Pastured butter (K2 source), grass-fed meats, pastured eggs, organic, pastured bacon, and coconut oil are preferred. All the hormones necessary for bone formation are derived from LDL cholesterol in our diet. Vegans should pay close attention to this biologic fact. Polyunsaturated fats and carbohydrates should be extremely limited during treatment to avoid future fractures because they generate inflammatory cytokines. Most

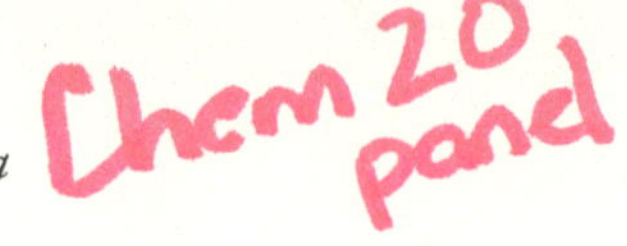

fructose and vegetable oils, which explains why the
s!

are not completely indicative of bone risk. I have had ralyzed from osteopenic fractures. Inflammation is ctor and should be followed clinically to assess risk. Bone density testing is worthless in my view unless a wrist module is added to it.

3. Smoking carries a 100-fold risk of developing osteoporosis. It must cease for any treatment to work! This is because smoking causes oxidized plasma. On a lipid profile you will see a very low HDL, an elevated HS-CRP, and low vitamin D. Smokers also show abnormal hormone panels.

4. Excessive alcohol use also elevates risk. More than 4 ounces of liquor a day is a problem. Excessive drinking causes low sodium (hyponatremia), a condition in the blood recently associated with the development of osteoporosis. It tends to cause bad balance and more frequent falls, and needs to be considered in the workup. This is easily picked up on the Chem 20 panel.

5. I personally avoid all conventional osteoporotic drugs because of the side effect risks. In surgical cases, I now completely avoid the use of all synthetic-derived bone morphogenic proteins in older patients with osteoporosis (Medtronic(r) InFuse for example).

6. I use high dose vitamin D3, K2, and magnesium in doses based on lab data and the severity of disease. I do not use calcium supplementation.

7. I replace all sex steroid hormones to the top quartile found in young adults using bio-identical hormone replacement therapy. I avoid synthetic hormones at all costs. Often this is tough because many physicians are not aware why synthetic hormones are suboptimal for the human steroid receptor. Medroxyprogesterone has a hydroxyl group in a position that normal progesterone does not. Evolution did not prepare for this situation and that is precisely why the Women' Health Initiative study was a total disaster. If bio-identical progesterone was used we likely would have gotten a different result-the result Europeans got when they studied this. Conventional medicine says synthetic equals bio-identical. I call bullshit on that. Watch Matt "The Kracken" LaLonde's video 2011 video, An Organic Chemist's

Perspective on Paleo, to see this statement supported by a Harvard-trained organic chemist.

8. Exercise is an excellent treatment for osteoporosis and is often underutilized. But with leptin resistance, exercise exacerbates the risk of fracture because Wolff's law is null and void. The Exercise Rx (written below) requires Wolff's law to be operational to work. Too often it is not. Exercise will increase growth hormone and testosterone secretion, which is very anabolic for bone mass accumulation. Most older people have horrendous growth-hormone levels measured by IGF-1 levels. In people with IGF-1 levels below 100, I recommend the use of arginine, ornathine, turmeric, and resveratrol because all increase bone mass. Resveratrol increases endogenous bone morphogenic proteins directly.

Walking is a great start for those who are debilitated. I tell my patients to park far away from doors to facilitate walking. I encourage water aerobics because it's low impact and has good skeletal effects, even when Wolff's law is null and void. I also encourage yoga and meditation for endogenous control of cortisol. Biofeedback is also a consideration if it is in the budget.

9. Strict avoidance of NSAIDs and steroids for all people with osteopenia or spine fusions due to bone mass losses. These medications also cause a leaky gut and promote gut dysbiosis, major causes of persistent inflammation and bone loss.

10. Any stressor should be aggressively treated. I usually double doses of D3, K2 and magnesium during ICU, preoperative times, or stressful life events such as death of a loved one, divorce, or a wedding.

11. In older patients, I trim back all medications that cause osteoporosis and advocate strongly for hormone replacement. Progesterone is critical for women and testosterone for men. Estrogen and testosterone are often added to women's treatment plan by their PCPs, or Ob/GYNs, or NPs.

12. I try to limit radiation exposure to all patients with osteopenia because of its effects on bone tissue.

13. I have all thoracic fracture patients follow up with their lung specialists because each fracture limits pulmonary functioning by 5-8 percent and is a major cause of pulmonary disability.

14. Any spine fracture should be aggressively treated surgically as soon as it is diagnosed on STIR MRI.

15. I keep an open dialogue with patients and family about bone risks and make sure they know what to discuss with their PCPs while going forward.

16. Mobility is the key to optimal recovery. We want patients moving naturally as soon as possible to stimulate bone formation after the diet is optimized.

17. I do not advocate the use of any calcium with this disease because I mandate a diet that provides ample calcium, so there is no need for supplementation. Calcium supplementation might be dangerous with a vitamin K2 deficiency and accounts for the morbidity and mortality data recently reviewed in the literature.

18. For severe cases I will ask for an endocrine consult to consider Forteo and PTH if it is warranted. This is quite rare but can be a huge help in complicated spine fractures in older patients.

19. I advocate sun exposure for natural vitamin D production in patients with low omega 6/3 ratios. This is outlined in my vitamin D blog on my website.

FALL PREVENTION AND THE EXERCISE RX FOR OSTEOPOROSIS

After you adopt a Paleolithic diet and deal with the underlying leptin resistance, everything should be done to prevent falls that can cause fractures. This is where exercise comes in. I am a major advocate of lifting weights for both men and women, no matter their baseline condition. If the patient is wheelchair bound they can lift dumbbells while they watch TV, and wear weighted ankle and wrist bracelets. The reason is simple. This will restore bone faster than any single thing we can offer once the dietary problem is repaired.

Also, men and women with osteoporosis need to take care not to fall down. Falls can break bones and are a major source of disability. Once mobility is limited the death rate can begin to grow exponentially. The goal is to restore natural mobility as soon as possible in this disease.

Some reasons people fall are:

- Poor vision
- Poor balance
- Certain diseases that affect how you walk
- Some types of medicine, such as sleeping pills

Some tips to help prevent falls outdoors are:

- Use a cane or walker
- Wear rubber-soled shoes so you don't slip
- Walk on grass when sidewalks are slippery
- In winter, put salt or cat litter on icy sidewalks

Some ways to help prevent falls indoors are:

- Keep rooms free of clutter, especially on floors
- Use plastic or carpet runners on slippery floors
- Wear low-heeled shoes that provide good support
- Do not walk in socks, stockings, or slippers
- Be sure carpets and area rugs have skid-proof backs or are tacked to the floor
- Be sure stairs are well lit and have rails on both sides
- Put grab bars on bathroom walls near tub, shower, and toilet
- Use a rubber bath mat in the shower or tub
- Keep a flashlight next to your bed
- Use a sturdy step stool with a handrail and wide steps
- Add more lights in rooms

Buy a cordless phone to keep with you so that you don't have to rush to the phone when it rings, and so that you can call for help if you fall.

REFERENCES

1. In fact in medical school we learned about Chvostek's and Trousseau's sign for calcium deficiency but they actually also tell us more about magnesium deficiency. I use these tests in osteoporosis and migraine patients daily. I see these more commonly in diabetics today than any other sign.
2. Chvostek's sign may also be present in hypomagnesemia, frequently seen in alcoholics, persons with diarrhea, patients taking aminoglycosides or diuretics, because hypomagnesemia can cause hypocalcemia. Magnesium is a cofactor for adenylate cyclase. Adenylate cyclase catalyzes the conversion of ATP to 3',5'-cyclic AMP. The 3',5'-cyclic AMP (cAMP), which is required for parathyroid hormone activation.

Chapter Seven

DISEASE TWO: OBESITY

THE PRIMAL RX MEETS THE LEPTIN RX-HOW TO PERFORM BRAIN SURGERY WITHOUT A SCALPEL

If you have read my blog, you will know that I cut my teeth writing about leptin in my Quilt Treatise online. Leptin was discovered in 1994, after I graduated from medical school, so I had never heard of it. I barely remember hearing about it in residency, when we had to cover hypothalamic biochemistry and pathophysiology. These are the talks that put neurosurgeons to sleep.

Leptin is a hormone with many evolutionary functions. It helps regulate hunger and appetite. It decides whether the liver burns glucose instead of fat through its ability to turn on or off PEPCK. PEPCK is an enzyme that regulates gluconeogenesis, the synthesis of glucose. From an evolutionary standpoint, leptin controls fertility and selects the immature egg cell in the ovary for fertilization every month. Any hormone that controls this critical step is clearly a main determinant in our species' overall biologic plan, as evolution selects for reproductive fitness. Leptin is also the master hormone that controls the action and release of all the other hormones made in the brain or the adrenal cortex, thyroid gland, and in the gut. When leptin goes, the other hormones go. Leptin is the conductor of the energy metabolism orchestra and the first hormone over which we must regain control to re-engineer a person back to his or her biologic potential.

Leptin also controls satiety in the brain. Elevated leptin signals the brain we have eaten enough. But when you eat too much, the brain becomes blind to its signal thanks to leptin resistance. Obesity leads to leptin resistance because leptin is in all fat cells and the fatter you are the more leptin you have. Leptin levels in the obese are usually above 10 ng/ml, whereas normal levels are 4-9 ng/ml. When leptin levels are under 4 ng/ml, we find people struggling with infertility and anorexia.

IS LEPTIN RESISTANCE A DISEASE OR A SYMPTOM? FIBROMYALGIA AND LYME DISEASE

The first time I saw Michelangleo's David in Florence, I went all around the statue to see the details of his anatomy cut into the carrera marble. I marveled at the amazing detail by a master sculptor, but something else struck me. Every picture you see of this statue is from the front or the side. This is what we have become conditioned to seeing. However, being in Florence helped me see the statue from a new perspective and I was fascinated with the oblique and back views of the statue. Later that night while I was looking at my photos of the sculpture, I looked down at my own morbidly obese body and a lightening bolt of insight struck me. What if I looked at obesity as a symptom instead of as a disease? Would that change the way I might help myself? It was that insight that led me to the science that underpins the Leptin Rx.

That night I searched the Internet to begin reconstructing the biochemical processes that determine fat storage. I then asked myself what was different about fat manufacture and fat storage in the statue's figure versus my own. I wanted to compare fat manufacturing and storage between a fit human and someone obese like myself. This insight forced me to look at epigenetic, genetic, environmental, biochemical, and hormonal factors as the real causes of obesity.

Leptin resistance alters brain signaling. This is caused by inflammation at the parts of the brain where leptin enters, the circumventricular (CV) organs. The most important CV for leptin is at the median eminence of the pituitary gland, which connects the pituitary gland with the hypothalamus. If leptin cannot enter, it cannot tell the brain what the energy status is of the body. This is like driving 80 mph from New York to Los Angeles with mud smeared across the windshield and a broken gas gauge. You will have no way of knowing how much gas you really have! That is leptin resistance in a nutshell.

If you run out of gas, you go nowhere, which is what happens in a disease such as fibromyalgia or Lyme disease. They both facilitate leptin resistance because both cause tremendous inflammation in the central nervous system, blocking leptin from doing its job. As another example, what would your world be like if you had no electricity, gasoline, coal, wind power, solar energy, geothermal energy, or nuclear energy? Let us take it further. What do we call a human body with no ability to produce energy? We call that person a cadaver. Leptin controls all energy production in the human body. It controls the entire hormonal response of the brain and all the signaling energy generation pathways in the body. Leptin is the kingpin.

So when we understand leptin's relationship to our cellular responses, we have the Rosetta Stone to understanding our body's byzantine biochemical reactions. Our leptin status and the resultant hormonal levels help us decipher our body's response to our environment and our diet. Trying to gauge this by following our diet or hormones alone is too difficult to decipher, but many people try. This also is not something modern medicine does. When you understand that evolution first checks with the hormones that control energy balance to decide whether we can reproduce, you begin to realize how incredibly important leptin really is. Diabetics are insulin resistant but they can have children. Those who are profoundly leptin resistant cannot have children. The same is true in experimental animals bred to be born without leptin. In fact, fertility experts now say one in eight couples in the United States are infertile. Do you think infertility clinics routinely screen those people for leptin resistance? They do not, but they should

WHO ARE PEOPLE WITH LEPTIN RESISTANCE?

Clinically, the two ends of leptin resistance are the morbidly obese and those with anorexia nervosa. Both are profoundly leptin resistant, but one has high leptin levels and the other has very low leption. One has huge energy stores (obese) and the other has none (anorexic). In between these two diseases are those with hypothalamic amenorrhea, fibromyalgia, Lyme disease, adrenal fatigue, chronic fatigue syndromes-in other words, those with burned-out cortisol levels and crashed sex steroid hormone levels. This is how a clinician who practices evolutionary medicine uses a patient's hormone status to determine what to do next. These diseases can all be cured when you open your mind to a new perspective.

EVOLUTIONARY MEDICINE AND THE PRIMAL RX

I believe we know less than 5 percent of what really controls our biologic processes today, as the system is very complex. But we need to ask how we can incorporate all new information with what we already know. That is a core Primal RX principle.

Most doctors know the individual biologic processes at work in our bodies, but not how they work together. I use this analogy with my patients: Say your wife told you she had an extra $250,000 and was going to buy the Ferrari you always wanted. She calls the Italian manufacturer and orders the car, getting it for only $200,000 because she bought it direct from the factory disassembled. You both smile when it comes to your house in 500 boxes. But now she says she wants to ride in it as soon as possible. You explain this is impossible because you need to find someone to put it together first. This is exactly what your doctor faces today. Doctors know all the parts of our biology, but they do not yet know how all these parts work together. That is the missing link in modern medicine.

IS THE PRIMAL RX THE KEY TO LONGEVITY?

I was totally blind to this fact until I injured myself and became a patient. My injury gave me an appreciation of how the Ferrari is assembled and how all the parts work together. For me, understanding how leptin fit in was key to understanding optimal health and Neolithic disease. Hormonal responses reflect how the brain responds to biochemical pathways that converge on our mitochondria. Our mitochondria are where energy is made or lost in every cell. If we are energy efficient, our cells respond by making adequate adenosine triphosphate (ATP), the energy currency of a cell, and by not shortening the telomeres on our chromosomes.

Telomeres are the ends caps on our chromosomes that determine how long a cell may live. It appears, based on the work of Elizabeth Blackburn, PhD at University of California, San Francisco, telomeres determine how well each organ in our body works and how long they will last us in our life. She won the Nobel Prize for her work in 2009. Since we know leptin is tied to telomere biology, we know it is important to optimal health and a long lifespan. We also know those who are leptin resistant are prone to many Neolithic diseases that cause them to get sick earlier and many have a shortened life span.

When I began my Leptin Reset, I did a telomere test and it gave me a biologic age older than my chronologic one. I retested myself two other times to see whether losing the weight lengthened my telomeres, and the test showed it did. The telomere test is a very rough estimate of cellular aging and has a seven-year margin of error. Nevertheless, I was happy to see losing weight was helping on a cellular level. I found it comforting that I could reverse engineer earlier mistakes in life. Telomere biology is the best stick to measure healthy lifestyle choices today in my opinion.

OBESITY IS THE MAJOR SYMPTOM OF MANY NEOLITHIC DISEASES

Obesity and its related disorders is the largest public health problem in America today. Two-thirds of Americans in 2011 were either overweight or obese. Obesity increases the risk of high blood pressure, diabetes, stroke and heart attack, making it the most significant health symptom in the United States. The surgeon general estimates more than 300,000 deaths are attributable to obesity each year. Obesity is tied to many secondary Neolithic diseases, such as sleep apnea, autoimmune disease, chronic infections, Lyme disease, candida overgrowth, fibromyalgia...the list goes on.

THE CONVENTIONAL WISDOM APPROACH RX OF OBESITY:

Apparently you practice gluttony and sloth routinely. You should eat less and exercise more! Oh yeah, you're really lazy and not motivated, too. You should count every calorie and do cardio until you puke. You need to go on a low-fat, high-carbohydrate diet advocated by the alphabet soup organizations under the American Medical Association, such as the ACA, ADA, and AHA.

None of this is good advice if you are obese or overweight. In fact, it is a guarantee you will stay fat and likely get fatter. This way you will be able to feed the health care system for its profit. You will see many physicians and be given a steady flow of medicines designed to treat your symptoms and not your underlying pathology. No one seems to have answer to cure obesity. Dr. Atkins had much success treating obesity with his diet, but the American Medical Association tried to take his license away from him for opposing its diet. The Atkins diet clearly has its flaws (high levels of omega six and the use of Neolithic toxins) but it was far superior to the SAD advocated by conventional medicine in terms of resolving Neolithic disease and obesity. Moreover, low-carb (below 100 grams) and high-fat diets outperform most diets in head-to-head research trials. Interestingly, this diet has not been tested against a ketogenic Paleolithic diet in a trial. This is something that should happen soon considering how many Americans are obese.

TOUCHED BY THE CONVENTIONAL WISDOM (CW) FAIRY?

What are the other clinical signs that you have been touched by the CW fair for obesity treatment?

I bet you are on at least five of these medicines:

- Statins
- Premarin
- Synthroid
- Prilosec
- Hydrocodone
- Norvasc
- Glucophage/metformin
- Albuterol
- Claritin
- Prozac
- Sleeping pills

This is a sure sign you have little hope of losing weight with your current treatment plan. Most of these drugs are given for symptoms caused by elevated cortisol level and disruption in the normal diurnal pattern of cortisol release. Obesity is associated with a chronic high cortisol, insulin resistance, and leptin resistance. I can say this as a previously morbidly obese patient myself, and as a physician who used these drugs to try and help people get to their goals. Epic failure is what one usually gets. Obesity is an inflammatory brain disorder, and until we treat it as such we will never conquer it.

WHAT IS THE OPTIMAL RX FOR OBESITY? THE LEPTIN RX RESET

This is precisely how I cured my family and myself of obesity. The neurobiology of obesity is vast, and much of it is still unknown. I do not claim to know the cure to obesity, but I know this path helps people get to a place where they can actually think about reaching their weight loss goals. Anyone who says they understand it all is lying or is unaware of how much we don't know yet. I do think, however, this protocol, which I developed after 20 years of training in multiple disciplines, works for many.

First, this protocol is how I cured myself of this problem. When people saw my results they asked me for the Rx. I was not sure this worked on everyone so I needed to try it on a few others to see if it could work for people of various ages and for both sexes. As proof, my first two patients to do this were a 16-year-old male (my son) and a 21-year-old male (my nephew), neither with any training in biology. As a formerly obese male myself, I had tried everything under the sun prior to taking matters into my own hand. Most obese people are wary of any new dietary advice because they have tried everything, too. I get it, trust me. There are no gimmicks here. We are using the tools evolution gave us to fix you. No drugs or fancy meal plans are needed. And forget counting calories. It is an epic waste of time that will only raise your cortisol due to the stress. When you begin this, you will be shocked at how your cravings and hunger go away for the first time in your life and don't come back. Moreover, you can control this forever if you choose. This is not a maybe, it's a lock. You don't need to know the biochemistry. You simply need to eat via leptin's biologic cycles as evolution dictated. Here is how one might consider doing it.

THE OPTIMAL RX FOR OBESITY: BRAIN SURGERY WITHOUT USING A SCALPEL.

1. First make sure you really are leptin resistant to begin with. The easiest way to do this is to look in the mirror. If you are obese or overweight by 25 pounds, you are leptin resistant. If you're broke, this is the easiest and cheapest way to assess your condition. If you're a tester like I am, you can draw some labs.

If you have a large appetite and crave foods, especially carbohydrates at night, you are likely leptin resistant. If you are fit or in decent shape and not sure based upon the above symptoms, get a blood test and check your:

- Reverse T3
- Leptin levels
- Salivary cortisol levels, or your
- Ferritin levels
- C-reactive protein

They all will be elevated to some degree. I also like to draw a highly sensitive C-reactive protein to gauge the level of inflammation. The higher this number is the longer your reset will take. The reason is simple. Obesity is an inflammatory brain disease, not one of gluttony or sloth.

I also recommend checking your salivary cortisol level because it is the key to knowing your situation. You will see either an overall elevation or cortisol or a spike during the wrong time of the day. A nighttime cortisol spike when it should be at its lowest is common with leptin resistance. A normal cortisol rhythm is highest in the morning and lowest in the evening. Leptin does the exact opposite and causes it to be low in the morning and high in the evening.

2. To regain leptin sensitivity follow a strict Paleolithic diet as outlined in The Paleo Solution by Robb Wolf or The Paleo Answer by Loren Cordain. You can use other books but these are my two go-to books for obese patients.

The type of fuel you eat is as important as is eliminating the foods that cause leptin receptors to become nonfunctional. These two books clearly outline a solid reference point to achieve this.

A. Try to eat as soon as possible in the morning, ideally within 30 minutes of waking. Make sure your breakfast has little to no carbs (less than 50 grams), and is rich in protein and fat. I use as a general rule 50-75 grams of protein with most patients. Some patients can use less and some need more. You'll know how much is right for you based on your hunger later in the day. If you remain ravenous throughout the day, you need to eat more protein in the morning. If you can hold off eating until dinner you probably are at homeostasis. If you can skip both meals you likely are overdoing it at breakfast. Try to go at least 4-5 hours between meals and before bed. As for sources, I suggest pastured or organic eggs first, served with leftover grass-fed meats, poultry, or fish from dinner. A third option, although less ideal, would be whey protein or protein shakes. I am not a fan of whey protein because it is a processed protein. I generally make breakfast from dinner because it's easy to take leftovers to the office.

B. Try to limit carbohydrate intake to 25 grams if you are overweight by more than 30 pounds. If you are fit and have a small amount of weight to lose, (less than 30 pounds) you can titrate up your carbs. Even then, I do not advocate potatoes or rice, which some Paleo diets allow while you are on the reset. The reset is temporary and not designed to be the way you will eat forever. (That will be covered in the Leptin PostRx discussed later in this chapter.) You will be able to eat these foods eventually, but try to avoid most starches until you have mastered your cravings and hunger. Do not count calories; it is not needed at this point. Any time I eat carbs I use liberal amounts of pastured butter, raw heavy cream, coconut, palm oil, or ghee. I do not recommend other oils initially, such as olive oils or industrial seed oils. I would also avoid nut oils at the initial stages. My personal favorite is coconut oil. It's medium-chain triglyceride (MCT) oil has great metabolic effects and helps heal the "leaky guts" of leptin-resistant folks.

3. How you eat your fuel is MORE IMPORTANT than any other factor, including the food itself. The Leptin RX is tied to circadian chronobiology. These rules are vital to follow for success.

A. Never snack. This means initially and forever. Snacking completely stresses the liver's metabolism. Your liver needs to relearn how to use gluconeogenesis when you are asleep and awake. Snacking destroys the timing and circadian clocks that work in unison with leptin. Once you synchronize leptin, all the other hormones that people struggle with tend to react well either with dietary changes or slight help from your doctor.

B. Try to eat three meals a day initially, but as your hunger and cravings fade you can adapt to two a day.

C. Try to eat breakfast as early as possible from rising. The sunrise is critical to re-yoking your circadian clocks once again.

D. Do not work out before or after breakfast. In obesity your cortisol is already high, so we don't want to drive it higher to cause a pregnenelone steal syndrome. This will cause adrenal fatigue, cause your sex steroid hormones to crater, and worsen your body composition.

E. Try to allow 4-5 hours between meals and sleep time.

F. If you decide to work out, do it after 5 p.m. to stimulate fat burning during sleep.

G. Within an hour of sunset try to make your surroundings as dark as possible.

H. If you have trouble falling asleep, I suggest 3-5 minutes of body weight exercises right before bed (pushups or air squats are fine, but avoid this if your evening cortisol is high on salivary cortisol testing).

I. If you're inclined, try becoming mindful when you first lay down. I use transcendental meditation techniques to help me clear my mind and concentrate on improving my thinking. (Optional; but this is awesome if your evening cortisol is high on your salivary testing).

4. Most people will notice a change in their cravings and hunger within 4-6 weeks. The higher your homocysteine and C-reactive protein, or the more underlying hormonal variability you have, the longer the Leptin Rx reset will take. There is no right time because everyone's inflammation levels vary. This means men in andropause and women in menopause will take longer for this to occur. I generally tell these patients they will be better off if they have their hormones optimized with bio-identical hormone therapy while doing the Leptin Rx reset.

I also advise my patients to supplement with prescription-grade fish oils and vitamin D3. The dose depends upon the homocysteine and C-reactive protein levels, vitamin D levels, and salivary cortisol levels.

5. Signs that you are becoming leptin sensitive again and that you should consider migrating to the Leptin Post Rx.

A. Men will notice quick weight loss.

B. Women will notice mood changes first (calmer or more sleepy) and their sleep will improve. Their clothes will fit differently but weight may not change drastically initially because of effects on the pituitary. Leptin is also a sexually dimorphic hormone, meaning it has different effects in men and women. This will change, too, if they continue moving forward.

C. You will notice a change in your sweating pattern.

D. You will notice you have better recovery from exercise and your energy levels seem to have risen.

E. Your hunger is gone and so are your cravings.

F. When you awaken you will feel very refreshed, like you slept well.

Generally when the signs are all present, I then really push high-intensity interval training (HIIT) exercise with heavy weights.

For more questions on the Leptin Rx, visit my website and look at the blog post called the Leptin Rx FAQs and How does the Leptin Rx work? The reader comment sections of these blogs contain gold. Under the nutrition tab at www.marksdailyapple.com there is a monster thread filled with awesome information and testimonials.

WHAT DO YOU DO ONCE THE LEPTIN RESET IS COMPLETE?

OK, so what do you do after you complete the reset and you want to continue toward optimal living? You transition to the Leptin Rx Postscript coming soon in this chapter. Follow this plan once you meet the clinical signs. This is precisely how I eat today without exception. Eating this way I have maintained a 135-pound weight loss with no issues at all.

The Leptin Rx causes the hypothalamus to respond to food in a new way by sensitizing the leptin receptor to account for electrons from food in the way evolution designed. In essence, we alter genetic expression by altering our diet and synchronizing it with light cycles. I describe it to my patients as, "performing brain surgery without a blade." When you adopt the Leptin Rx, the organs' responses are dramatically different. They send new messages to the brain via the vagus nerve, which happens in 6 to 8 weeks for most people. These changes can be followed by the clinician or the patient and are outlined in the Leptin FAQ blog post on my website:

Changes in appearance: Your hair and nails will improve in color and presentation. Your pedicurist will notice you have less dead skin on your feet. Your face will look a better, with softer skin and better color, especially if you use olive oil or coconut oil on your skin.

Changes in mood, personality, and thoughts: You will become more thoughtful, more mindful, and less explosive. If you decide to add mindfulness to your reset (you should), you will notice tremendous changes in your thinking and your ability to learn and comprehend. Your insight, intuition, and mental acuity will sharpen. Also, your sexual desires will change and your libido will awaken. Your spouse will begin to notice and treat you differently.

Changes in appetite: Your carbohydrate cravings will go away. You'll feel full and not really need to eat three meals a day. You'll notice your taste and smell change.

Changes in energy and sleep: Over 6-12 months, expect your energy to gradually improve. You will feel warmer and exude body heat, but your body temperature will actually be lower. It will continue to trend lower over the next 18-24 months while you thyroid settles into its new biologic groove. Dramatic improvements will be made in your sleep. Both migraines and muscle soreness from exercise will decrease.

The Leptin Reset forces the brain to see signals that confuse the leptin receptors. The brain's response is to revert to an older known pathway. I am using past neurobiology research here. For instance, the neuroscientist Michael Merzenich, PhD was able to figure out a way to allow deaf people to hear again by stimulating the auditory cortex of the brain. By giving this area of the brain a signal, the brain relearned how to hear. This is how the cochlear implant was born. Other information that helped me create the Leptin Rx came from the neuroscientist Vilayanur Ramachandran, PhD and his work curing phantom limb pain with a mirror. Ramachandran found using a mirror to reflect the image of the existing limb tricked the brain into thinking the amputated limb was still there. Then the patient could work on relaxing the limb to manage the pain.

This is an example of how one does not need expensive technology to induce gene expression. It is possible to do without an NIH grant, too. It requires thought, clinical experience, and a basic understanding of how the brain works. Evolution designed the brain to decipher puzzles so we can learn and manage our environment. My Leptin Rx reset process uses the same principles to help obese patients get back to optimal. That is the essence of the Leptin Rx reset-brain surgery without a scalpel.

We can force the hypothalamus to once again rely on circadian and ultradian (ultradian means occuring regularly throughout the day) rhythms during the Leptin Rx reset process. We can use lab testing to show the leptin receptor has regained its ability to yoke to meal timing and light cycles. We induced this gene expression by forcing the change. It has nothing to do with laziness or with gluttony. Obesity is an inflammatory brain disease. When the brain is faced with confounding sensory variables it reverts to evolutionary standbys. The circadian cycles are among the oldest biologic rhythms found in all life forms on earth, something the brain knows well and depends on.

These biologic responses are already built into our DNA and waiting to be used. Until now, no one really looked for it. I use the allegory that evolution is like the North Star, always there, never moving, and a source that people might use to keep their direction focused upon weight loss without much effort.

WHAT IF I AM ALREADY AT A GOOD WEIGHT AND I JUST NEED TO GET A BETTER BODY COMPOSITION?

Now we are going to talk about how one might consider eating and living after the reset is complete. This method is where a Paleo or primal person who is already fit and healthy may consider starting. If you simply want to look better naked or in a bikini, start here. It optimizes our biologic clocks and rhythms for optimal performance and body composition when performed consistently over time.

WHAT IF MY VAGUS NERVE WAS CUT BY SURGERY?

The solution for you is to add my cold thermogenesis protocol listed on my blog at http://jackkruse.com/the-evolution-of-the-leptin-rx/. Read how to add cold thermogenesis to enhance success. And when we get to the last chapter of this book you will begin to see why cold thermogenesis is major benefit to all mammals.

THE LEPTIN RX POSTSCRIPT

1. Plan on eating a straightforward primal/Paleo template as outlined in the those books mentioned in Chapter Three. If you are very active you can add carbohydrates from 10-30 percent of your diet. The diet is still a high-fat, moderate-protein Paleo template outlined in the Paleo books.

2. Within one hour of rising, eat 50 percent of your daily carbs with 25 grams of protein and 20-30 grams of fat.

3. Never miss breakfast because it stimulates the circadian rhythm for gastric acid secretion in adults. This will become critical later in the day for body composition optimization.

4. Avoid working out prior to breakfast. It is a circadian cycle breaker because it raises cortisol at a time it is already high.

5. For optimal results, you must get most of your daily activity between 9 a.m. and 4 p.m. when light cycles are strong year round. This is another reason I strongly advocate high vitamin D levels year round. We evolved around the equator and the equatorial sun has been shown to keep human vitamin D levels at between 50-150 ng/mL. Avoid sitting at all costs and consider walking to get lunch or a short run during your midday break. The real goal here is to increase non-exercise activity thermogenesis (NEAT) during strong light hours. This has major effects when done consistently over time. For example, I avoid elevators and run upstairs and I park far away from my destinations to increase my NEAT daily. I also carry all my groceries out to the car and never use a shopping cart to make it easier. I look at every aspect of my actions to make sure I am maximizing it for NEAT.

6. For lunch, if you need to eat it (some won't eventually), you should consider eating 25 percent of your remaining daily carbs. I use this meal as a snack now. Rarely is it a big meal for me any longer. If I am intermittent fasting, this is the meal I cut like a bad habit. If you want more information on intermittent fasting, please visit Leangains.com or www.precisionnutrition.com/intermittent-fasting/summary.

7. Critical point: The best time to work out biologically occurs when it is least likely to be convenient for you because our Neolithic lives won't allow for it. I re-tooled my entire schedule as a surgeon to make this work optimally for me to lose weight and change my body. The ideal workout window is from 1-5 p.m. For best results, try to do the exercise in bright outdoor sunlight.

8. Dinner should be eaten within 45 minutes to 1 hour of this late afternoon work out. If you are leptin sensitive you can eat dinner this early and go comfortably without eating until breakfast the next day. During dinner you want to make sure to include a lot of protein (25-75 grams), the remainder of your carb allotment, and the balance in fats. The type of fats at dinner are also critical but are typical in a primal template. Try to concentrate on 10-18 carbon fatty acids because these are best at stimulating cholecystokinin (CCK), which destroys the nighttime appetite. I use coconut oil, ghee, pastured butter, and bacon lard to get this effect. I use the fat to cover the carbs and the protein most times in sauces.

9. Try to complete dinner by 7 p.m. This is critical in autumn and winter for optimal results. Eight p.m. is the outer limit for dinner in spring and summer. I actually alter my meal times very precisely as the light cycle changes during the year. Many people might find this too regimented. I agree but I do it because I had to make a huge clinical move to come down from 44 percent body fat. By strictly following this my first year I lost 133 pounds in 11 months. So the small details make a huge difference in good results versus optimal results.

10. Get to sleep by 11 p.m. in spring and summer months. I stay up longer June 10th to July 10th due to summer solstice on June 21. During this time of the year, I tend to have higher body fat with longer light cycles. In autumn and winter when the clocks are set back one hour stice I am in bed by 10 p.m. I have found I am leanest during this time of the year just like most wild animals are. Most humans who eat a SAD at their own convenient times will notice they get fattest in the winter months. This is when people make New Year's Resolutions, too, although few keep them.

The sleep goal is an optimal 7.5-8 hours a night, no matter the season. You will know when you are doing well because you will no longer need an alarm clock and your sleep wake cycle will be automatic. I found after one year of using this protocol I no longer needed an alarm clock to wake up for surgery.

WHAT CHANGES SHOULD I CONSIDER AFTER THE LEPTIN RX RESET?

1. If you are active, drop all of the top 10 Paleo supplements I mentioned that one might consider when doing the Leptin Rx reset. For this list you can visit my website at http://www.jackkruse.com/what-are-the-top-ten-paleo-supplements/. They were only meant for the transition from a sugar-burning to a fat-burning metabolism as the Paleo template takes flight. If you are not active, I would strongly consider you remain on pyrroloquinoline quinone and vitamin D3. Try to optimize your vitamin D levels to 60-100 ng/mL all year long. I prefer natural sunlight over a vitamin D3 supplement. I use the current omega-6 to omega-3 ratio as my guide when to push natural sunlight over a supplement. When your ratio is below 4:1 you can get sunlight without worrying much about skin cancer generation. I do not buy into the conventional wisdom that all sunlight is sinister no matter the context.

2. If you decide to do intermittent fasting, try not to skip breakfast. This often goes against most varieties of intermittent fasting protocols, but I stand by my recommendations because of the circadian biology of gastrin. I think you can try other methods and see the results you get. Do the one that works best for you. Eating a protein-laden breakfast is the key to circadian congruity and optimal body composition. You will see below how this determines body composition, not the amount of exercise one does.

KEY POINTS TO KEEP IN MIND ABOUT POST LEPTIN RX CHANGES:

1. High protein consumption occurs at night now, not at breakfast as it did in the Leptin Rx reset. The reason is because late afternoon is when the human body is normally programmed to undergo upregulation of protein synthesis biochemically. This is how our biology is designed by God or evolution. If you remember, earlier I told you to eat half your carbs and a small protein load (about 25 grams) to prime the gastric acid circadian cycle for maximal effect later in the day. This is precisely the reason why. Gastric pH should be highest when we are eating our biggest protein load of the day, while simultaneously upregulating protein synthesis in our body. This maneuver actually influences our body composition more than any exercise could, if it were added to the equation at all. Doing this on time is akin to an orchestra playing in unison. It is a huge point to try to follow daily.

2. Carbohydrate consumption should parallel activity and light cycles. I often hear many in the primal world talk about carbs and activity. They always forget about the light cycle. If you are very active and work out more than four days a week in sunlight, you can handle 30 percent of your calories from carbs. If not, consider a 10-20 percent range. The closer I get to June 21st, the more carbs I eat, and as I move closer to Dec 21st, I am at a zero-carb diet. I give this to you as a baseline to work from. It is not meant for you to copy exactly as I do.

3. Exercise or physical activity is biologically optimal for us between 9 a.m. and 4 p.m. I understand this might be hard to fit into your schedule, but the payoff is massive. Let me explain why now. Remember that cortisol is highest in the morning to allow us to wake up. If you exercise before breakfast, you risk elevating your cortisol even higher. This will cause a pregnenolone steal syndrome, ruining the hormonal response that controls your lean muscle mass and fat ratios, and eventually your body composition.

If you continue to do this over time, it will slow the protein synthesis that occurs later in the afternoon and evening. Moreover, It will also ruin your sleep cycle (checked by having low DHEA levels) and you risk being in an overtrained situation. I think this is the biggest error I see in the primal community. My advice is don't even try it.

4. You achieve optimal protein synthesis if exercise occurs between 1-4 p.m. Make sure you're lifting days occur on the days of the week you can accomplish this. Save sprinting for days this won't work for your schedule. Use common sense about building this into your own life. Optimize your schedule to benefit your body composition. If you fight this trend you can still get ripped, but you will exhaust your stem cells in doing so and will lose years on the back end of your life. Timing is that important!

5. To show you how important timing meals to the light cycles is to humans, consider the following facts. If you are able to workout in the evening 30-45 minutes before your protein dinner, you actually triple the amount of protein synthesis that occurs compared to those who do not. This is how a hunter-gatherer attained an optimal body composition without having to do huge amounts of exercises. Moreover, if this is also yoked to the light cycle in winter when temperatures are below 40 degrees Fahrenheit, you can increase protein synthesis to 400 percent while tripling fat burning. This allows you to increase fat burning to shed more body fat faster while increasing lean muscle mass. NASA uses this technology for the astronauts who space walk. They discovered this data from the Sherpas, who help foreigners scale the last 2,000 feet of Mount Everest. This is also precisely why I am leanest around December 21st. At this time, light and temperature are at their lowest, so exercising in this window is the easiest way I know to shed body fat and gain muscle mass quickly. I went from 44 percent body fat to 19 percent in one year doing this.

When do we see ads in the newspapers for weight loss aids? The answer is January. Why? Because humans tend to get fat in winter. Now think about wild animals you see on the Discovery Channel. When are they leanest? In winter, when food is scarce and they have to forage for food in subzero temperatures. Most humans live biologically incongruent to how we were designed to live. We think it is perfectly fine to eat cakes, pies, and drink eggnog during six weeks of low light during the holidays. Well, it's not.

Once I thought about the leptin receptor biology and how I could reset it using circadian rhythms, I went back to my veterinarian friends and the exercise literature (Frank Booth) to figure how to live the rest of my life optimally and regain my optimal body form and metabolism. This is precisely how I live today. Feel free to call my operating room team and ask them when was the last time they ever saw me operating between 2 p.m. and 5 p.m. For the last five years the answer is never.

6. The high-protein and high-fat meals we eat at dinner diminish our appetite tremendously, allowing leptin released from the fat cells to enter the hypothalamus from midnight to 2 a.m. This sends messenger chemicals to the thyroid to burn excess fat. Sleeping is the second critical way in which we increase our body composition. We use sleep to get rid of excess fat and calories, using T3, leptin, and uncoupling proteins. During sleep, protein synthesis also occurs during the process of autophagy, when we recycle all our proteins that we used during the day. Sleep deprivation leads to increased levels of the inflammatory compounds IL-6 and TNF alpha, which simultaneously lowers our DHEA levels. Decreased sleep also blocks the secretion of growth hormone at night, which leads to increased abdominal fat and eventually decreased lean muscle mass. This is why patients with sleep apnea have terrible body composition as a rule. The lowered growth hormone leads to high nighttime cortisol release. This is why so many obese, leptin-resistant patients with sleep apnea feel the need to eat carbohydrates at night. Cortisol is supposed to spike in the morning when we wake up, not during sleep. People who wake up with high cortisol levels will also crave a lot of carbohydrates at breakfast. If this occurs chronically, it will diminish the gastric acid cycle and destroy our naturally occurring cycle for developing our ideal body composition.

Why does this occur? Cortisol stimulates the release of ghrelin, a gastric hormone that increases insulin. Ghrelin is an appetite stimulant and increases our drive to eat when we wake up. It is usually high when we wake up, or it spikes anytime cortisol is too high. Elevated cortisol is a constant feature of obesity. Cortisol should never be high during sleep. When ghrelin levels increase 30 percent from baseline, this drives carbohydrate cravings while decreasing leptin uptake in the brain by 50 percent. Elevated triglycerides and high inflammatory cytokines further block the action of leptin at the hypothalamus. This is commonly seen in metabolic syndrome and is an epidemic in the western world today. Evolution never naturally selected for this because it was not possible before the human brain evolved to where it is today. For leptin to enter the brain, ghrelin levels must be low.

This is why four to five hours after dinner is the best time for leptin to enter the brain. So if you do shift work, you must be a great sleeper and run on a ketogenic primal diet to have any chance for good body composition. I have met only one person in my life who did this.

This is how I help people lose weight using the Primal Rx. If you want more information or have questions about this please visit my website at www.jackkruse.com or visit www.marksdailyapple.com and visit the nutrition forum and look at the monster thread there that really is the first Primal Rx textbook for primal medicine. It's there and it's free, loaded with a ton of primal healthcare hacks. You will find a lot more information on many diseases in both places.

REFERENCES

1. http://www.nature.com/nature/journal/v226/n5252/abs/2261261a0.html
2. Moore JG, Halberg F. Circadian rhythm of gastric acid secretion in active duodenal ulcer: chronobiological statistical characteristics and comparison of acid secretory and plasma gastrin patterns with healthy subjects and post-vagotomy and pyloroplasty patients. Chronobiology International. 1987;4:101-110.
3. Moore JG, Merki H. Gastrointestinal tract. In: Physiology and Physiology of Biological Rhythms. Peter H. Redfern and Bjorn Lemmer, Editors. Berlin, Springer, 1997, pp.351-373.
4. Haus E. and Smolensky M.: Development of circadian time structure and blood pressure rhythms. In: Portman R.J., Sorof J.M., Inglefinger J.R. (eds). Clinical Hypertension and Vascular Disease: Pediatric Hypertension. Humana Press Inc., NJ, pp 45-73, 2004.
5. Haus E., Nicolau G., Lakatua D.J., Sackett-Lundeen L.: Reference values for chronopharmacology. Ann. Rev. Chronopharm. 4:333-342, 1988.
6. Rivkees S.A. and Hao H.: Developing circadian rhythmicity. Seminar in Perinatology 24(4):232-242, 2000.
7. Sara Mednick , Ken Nakayama, Jose L. Cantero, Mercedes Atienza, Alicia A. Levin, Neha Pathak & Robert Stickgold (2002). The restorative effect of naps on perceptual deterioration. Nature Neuroscience, published online May 28, 2002
8. Aeschbach D, Matthews JR, Postolache TT, Jackson MA, Giesen HA, Wehr TA (1999). Two circadian rhythms in the human electroencephalogram during wakefulness. American Journal of Physiology, 277, R1771-9
9. Meneses Ortega S, Corsi Cabrera M (1990). Ultradian rhythms in the EEG and task performance. Chronobiologia, 17, 183-94
10. Rector RS, Uptergrove GM, Morris EM, Borengasser SJ, Laughlin MH, Booth FW, Thyfault JP, Ibdah JA., Daily exercise vs. caloric restriction for prevention of nonalcoholic fatty liver disease in the OLETF rat model., Am J Physiol Gastrointest Liver Physiol. 2011 May;300(5):G874-83. Epub 2011 Feb 24.PMID:21350190

11. Bjorntorp P. 2001 Do stress reactions cause abdominal obesity and co-morbidities? Obesity Reviews 2: 73-86.

12. Cota, D et al. 2006 Hypothalamic mTor signaling regulates food intake. Science 312:927-930.

13. Woo,R. et al. 1982 Effect of exercise on spontaneous calorie intake in obesity. Amer. Journal of Clin. Nut. 36: 447-47

14. http://www.ted.com/talks/view/lang/en//id/184

15. http://www.jbc.org/content/272/44/27758.full.pdf

16. http://img52.imageshack.us/img52/9496/image107b.jpg

Chapter Eight

DIABETES: A DISEASE OF THE MODERN AGE

LEPTIN RESISTANCE CAUSES DIABETES.

Modern medicine considers diabetes a disease. I do not. I consider it a biologic mismatch created by modern life. We must remember diabetes has many correlations to poor health, including, but not limited to, disordered signaling and imbalanced circadian rhythms, genetic and epigenetic triggers, environmental toxins, and diets high in PUFAs and carbohydrates. The latter is especially problematic if the carbohydrates are fried or cooked at high temperatures in PUFAs, as they generate a toxic compound called acrylamide.

CONVENTIONAL ADVICE GIVEN TO A TYPE 2 DIABETIC

You eat way too many carbs. In fact, your excess eating caused you to put on excess fat, and your excess fat is what made you diabetic. That about covers it.

We will send you to a nutritionist or a dietician who will give you an American Diabetes Association diet, which will never cure your diabetes but instead make you medical annuity for the next 50 years. You will slowly get sicker from many diseases, for which your doctor will give you prescriptions. The longer you have diabetes, the sicker you will become. Eventually you will die from a chronic Neolithic disease associated with diabetes. If you have really bad lifestyle habits, you will get Alzheimer's disease and be put in a nursing home while Medicare empties out your life savings to pay for your care. You will be on so many medications your head will spin, and you will wind up on insulin, which eventually will kill you.

WHAT DIABETES REALLY IS

I believe diabetes is caused by humans eating carbohydrates 24/7 and relying on modern conveniences instead of facing a true winter like mammals are supposed to. In fact, I think our brain rapidly evolved because of a sped-up epigenetic program due to Factor X (more about that in the last chapter), and this allowed us to reduce normal hibernation down to two hours within our sleep cycle to control autophagy . This system has little room for error. When we eat outside our circadian rhythm it causes the entire system to misfire and diabetes is the result. Sound hard to believe?

Many scientists today believe the light cycle has the most important impact on our circadian biology and metabolism. Light cycles are important to all life, but most researchers are apparently unaware that mammals have an innate ability to change their internal clocks when their environment changes. When it's cold, humans stop using light cycles to yoke metabolism to sleep. We have an epigenetic switch that stops the suprachiasmatic nucleus, the part of the brain that generates a 24-hour rhythm, from using light when it is cold. This is because light cycles are not important in the freezing cold because carbohydrates cannot grow in the cold. Evolution alerts mammals to the changing seasons through temperature, not light. However, this alert no longer happens for modern man, who eats carbs 24/7 and doesn't endure much of winter's cold. We have warm clothes, energy-efficient houses, heated cars, and exposure to LED computer and television screens at night. These things elevate inflammatory cytokines, causing leptin resistance. I explain the complex biochemistry in my cold thermogenesis series on my blog, with cites included. But for now, I want you to be aware of this metabolic trap. Its mere presence is shocking enough, but its implications are far greater for modern humans with respect to diabetes.

Many say the introduction of artificial light altered our ability to sense light and dark. I think most people are aware of the degree to which circadian mismatches destroy metabolic function, laying the foundation for diseases. If you're diabetic, this knowledge is critical.

A circadian mismatch causes the slow erosion of the autophagy process. The autophagy process repairs and recycles proteins while we sleep, which extends life. Reduced autophagy leads to heart failure. Diabetics usually have sleep apnea, which causes poor autophagy and a lowered DHEA level. Biologic mismatches are best measured in animals by looking at heart failure and poor sleep. For humans, the rates of both are staggering. We got so smart so fast that we controlled our environment to the point of our genetic detriment by disrupting the autophagy process.

When one looks at the biochemistry of sleep and truly understands the power of autophagy for longevity, it becomes apparent that perhaps sleep is our primordial condition, not wakefulness. If I am correct, we evolved consciousness over time. In extreme cold environments, the process of autophagy becomes "super sensitized" to save energy while increasing our metabolic capabilities. In a TED talk, sleep researcher Jessa Gamble said humans living in dark, deep, cold shafts for a study became more energized and productive. In fact, they improved so much most wanted to go back to living in shafts after the study. Why? Cold, dark environments sensitize the human autophagy process without us actually having to sleep at all! This is something we can't do in long light cycles. Diabetics never enter this pathway, which is why they are always energy-depleted and tired. To achieve sensitive autophagy in light, we have to sleep well. Diabetics can't. This is an example of how metabolism and biochemistry can rewire in cold and dark environments. Diabetics need winter more than they know.

In fact, sleep is heavily selected for in cold, having influenced the design of mammalian nervous systems by evolution. This is why mammals can sleep so long underground in sub-zero temperatures and survive.

RADICAL RULE #1: A RADICAL RULE ABOUT SLEEP

Sleep and cold environments were our ancestors' primordial condition, and hence the starting point for life on our planet.

If we assume this to be true, it explains why epigenetics-outside influences on gene expression-is the dominant player. I think evolution used epigenetics to pass environmental information to succeeding generations. In the cold, our cell cycle slows down. To compensate, epigenetics speeds up.

Life at its genesis was likely static. To get the nutrients it needed, an organism used passive diffusion, which allows compounds in the surrounding environment to pass through the membrane. This manner of nutrient collection is highly inefficient, but the sensitivity of autophagy in cold made this process biologically plausible for much of evolutionary history. However, in order to improve access to nutrients, it appears organisms evolved into wakefulness to obtain them, using sleep for autophagic repair. Yes, you read that correctly.

I believe this metabolism remains in every organism today. If you ask sleep researchers (I have), they have told me this is a correct assumption. Because of this, I believe that sleep and autophagic processes are highly conserved across all species on our planet. We have yet to find a species that does not sleep at least some of the time. I think as wakefulness evolved, life moved from a static model to a dynamic one. Now you see why autophagy sits at position 15 on the Quilt on my website. It is a critical component of optimal living in all species, not just our own. And it is badly damaged in diabetes.

This also signals the coupling of movement to memory. Even today, all learning in higher-order animals is directly coupled to movement in their environment. The more one moves the more intelligent one becomes. I explained that in a February of 2012 blog article called, Are Starches Really Safe?. Diabetics often have cognitive impairments and suffer from higher rates of Alzheimer's disease and other neurodegenerative disorders. I believe this all is tied to altered cell membrane signaling from carbohydrates and from poor autophagy.

Researchers currently assume the only way a mammal can change its fatty acid concentration is through its diet. However, the PLoS ONE article "Changes in 'Good' Fatty Acid Concentration of Inner Organs Might Be Largely Independent of Diet" shows that n-6 polyunsaturated fatty acids (those with the final double bond at the sixth position) in cell membranes increases dramatically before the start of hibernation in marmots. This is to prepare the body, and particularly the heart, to function at very low temperatures. The transition to a higher content of n-6 fatty acids in membranes takes place rapidly just before the animals enter hibernation. The changes are reversed, again very quickly, at the termination of hibernation in spring, when the animals return to higher body temperatures. During both these periods the animal's food is unavailable as it is buried under snow, so it is a mechanism that happens independently of immediate diet.

What surprised the researchers was that the n-6 fatty acids are transported preferentially over other fatty acids, and the mechanism remains a mystery. The research also suggests the changes come from an internal clock, as the animals are isolated from environmental cues while hibernating deep underground.

Let's examine why evolution may have allowed mammals to do this.

The stimulus for hibernation in eutherian (placental) mammals is tied to high dietary carbohydrate intake (proven fact already in science and not controversial) and transfer of omega six into cell membranes prior to hibernation. This was not known until this article came out. The stimulus of plentiful dietary carbohydrates is a metabolic sign that they should soon den, fat and happy. This metabolic signal seems to change the fatty acid synthase (FAS) enzyme in the mammalian gut lining. FAS is crucial for the production of lipids and is regulated by insulin. People with diabetes or insulin resistance have defects in FAS. Also, studies show mice without the enzyme in their intestines develop chronic gut inflammation, which is a powerful predictor of insulin resistance. This biology is now coming to light in humans and you can read about it in my second cite. It appears all the biology is lining up quite well with my theory.

IS DIABETES AN EVOLUTIONARY ADAPTATION FOR SURVIVAL?

Why would evolution signal a mammal to replace its own cell membranes with PUFAs? Why should we pay attention to it? Because it has major implications for modern humans, who are direct descendants of these animals. Moreover, this evolutionary design allows for the potential development of an interesting conundrum. It appears the incorporation of PUFAs into cell membranes is a normal signal for mammalian hibernation. After all, mammals evolved in earth's polar environments. I also learned from organic chemistry that high concentrations of PUFAs in the cell membrane makes them very fluid in cold environments so they don't freeze. It is a cellular antifreeze. I also found out from Canadian frog biology that high glucose levels also act as an antifreeze for animals in extreme environments. If our cell membranes are filled with monounsatured fats (MUFAs) and saturated fats, they become too stiff to work in cold environments. This is an important mechanism as all organ function depends on proper cellular signaling.

These revelations led me to a shocking insight. Could diabetes be an ancient epigenetic program for survival, and not a disease after all?

Why would we need diabetes to survive? Then the answer occurred to me. I call it Factor X, which I explain in the last chapter. I checked my facts and continue to connect more dots. Diabetes is required in mammals, which are designed to adapt to cold environments.

Maybe, just maybe, it has become thought of as a Neolithic disease in humans because our ability to control our environment has dismissed our need to hibernate. After all, we know evolution is moving today faster than our genome can adapt, as many researchers have pointed out many times

Remember, we still have our mammalian Paleolithic genes, which control our use of carbohydrates and the up-regulation of PUFAs in our cell membranes. What is not so obvious, however, is that our brain's evolution has outpaced our biology, creating a mismatch in this system. As a result, we view diabetes as a disease when it is an evolutionary novelty created by our own rapid evolution.

This is how I see diabetes today. The skeptics will jump down my throat and point out that type 1 diabetes is a genetic disease. I think type 1 and 1.5 diabetes (slow onset type 1 diabetes) are decidedly epigenetic phenomena of this evolutionary mismatch. Epigenetics has sped up. This is why humans have no ability to stop diabetes once it starts, unless they get themselves into a cold environment. It is also why modern medicine has no cure, and why it remains a revolving-door disease filled with wallet biopsies and an increasing number of ineffective medications.

Friends have asked, "If this is not a disease, then how does nature cure diabetes on its own?" Well, can you cure a disease that is not a disease to begin with?

Insulin resistance expands fat to store the carbohydrates we ate during the long light cycles of summer. The process to reverse this system is hibernation in freezing cold. But since we no longer hibernate, you need to consider how you eat carbohydrates within the light cycles. Maybe what you thought was safe really isn't.

Cold is what completely reverses insulin resistance in mammals, and wakes them up when conditions are better for life. Humans abandoned this ability in our evolutionary history because we control our environment regardless of the temperature, but we still have the hibernation mechanisms within us. If we eat outside those mechanisms we get modern-day diabetes-we can eat all day year round, or we can eat a banana from Chili in the dead of winter in the Arctic Circle. Do you think evolution has a plan for these circumstances yet? No, it does not, and diabetes is the answer.

The result is we have created a world where we can eat carbohydrates and PUFAs 24/7, but can no longer access evolution's solution for insulin resistance. It also makes sense why we have no hard-wired metabolic pathways for fat removal. But cold thermogenesis does it remarkably well. This implies our ancestors' Paleolithic genes remained dominant as we evolved out of the savannas of Africa. It could even mean that other assumptions we have made are also wrong. We must realize that because our brain's development was so rapid in a short time frame, it allowed evolution to dismiss the ability in us to hibernate. It is clear the modern human diet creates the mismatch that is diabetes today.

RADICAL RULE #2

Evolution speeds up as time progresses. This is a known biologic fact. The faster evolution occurs, the greater our dietary mismatches become, and real causes of diabetes are revealed. Factor X, which is covered in the last chapter, is the reason.

RADICAL RULE #3

Epidemics are not caused by genetics. This is also a medical fact, but you would never get that from reading the literature on diabetes today.

THE EPI-PALEO RX FOR DIABETES

Do everything opposite of what the nutritionist, dietitian, or most physicians tell you, and keep it to yourself. When they hand you prescriptions, fold them, put them in your pocket, and use the money to buy one of the Paleo 1.0 diet books I recommended. You are probably laughing right now, but if you call my father-in-law or my own wife, they will tell you that is precisely what I asked them to do. I am a neurosurgeon, not an endocrinologist, so if I can do it for my own family, so can you. The hardest part for them was believing me. I had to write a special blog post just for my father-in-law so he could get it right. My wife was a three-year-long skeptic until she was diagnosed with type 2 diabetes, a disease that ran in her family. She was shocked she got it because she had none of the classic risk factors. She is an example of the epigenetic links that govern how diabetes is transmitted in mammals. We are importing this disease all over the world through bad nutritional advice and environmental toxins.

After about six months of battling with me, my wife finally gave up all grains and dairy (her nemesis), adopted a Paleolithic diet, and cured herself.

In fact, she never went back to see the physician who diagnosed her. I have found it harder to convince my immediate family than my patients of how this all works. They just can't fathom how easy it is to do. My diabetic patients have been so beaten down by medical mismanagement that by the time they come to me with a disc herniation or osteoporosis, they are ready to walk on hot coals when I tell them I can "treat" their diabetes. Cold thermogenesis is critical for all diabetics. The protocol is listed on my website at www.jackkruse.com/the-evolution-of-the-leptin-rx/.

Most type 2 diabetics are obese and most type 1 diabetics are not. I believe epigenetics is the real culprit here. Most type 1.5 diabetics (delayed onset autoimmune diabetes) are mixed due to the autoimmune nature of their diabetes. Diabetes has many causes in my opinion, but most cases are linked to a leaky gut at some level and a circadian rhythm mismatch. For the obese type 2 diabetics, I use the Leptin Rx with cold thermogenesis on them first, and try to get them to an optimal dietary template as fast as possible. For the ones, like my wife, who are not overweight, we use a very short course of the Leptin Rx and then switch them to the Leptin Rx Postscript diet, but use a ketogenic version of the Paleolithic diet until fasting blood glucose normalizes. Once that occurs, we transition them to diet that includes some carbohydrates. Not all can do this, but some can. I believe the answer lies within the brain's cell membranes, where signaling is broken by inflammatory cytokine storms. My best guess based on my current knowledge is that there is permanent loss of hypothalamic hypocretin neurons, which regulate sleep, wake, and appetite, and it alters the entire system's functionality.

A fasting blood sugar below 88 tells me leptin sensitivity is occurring at the liver level and the patient has regained control over gluconeogenesis, the synthesis of glucose. One thing that most diabetics struggle with, even when their HBA1c is good, is an inability to attain a fasting blood glucose below 88. Many articles call this the "dawn syndrome," a condition in which morning blood sugar is high. I call it, "someone who is late to the leptin party." If you fix leptin resistance, your fasting blood sugar will drop below 88 once again. The enzyme that regulates gluconeogenesis in humans is phosphoenolpyruvate carboxykinase (PEPCK). Guess what controls this enzyme? LEPTIN!!!! So once you fix leptin, you fix the vexing issue of high morning blood sugar. The best way to fix leptin has already been covered in the Leptin Reset chapter.

The Epi-paleo Rx works for all types of diabetics, even type 1. It will not cure true type 1 diabetes, but it will make you healthier because it is so anti-inflammatory. The diet also works for those with type 1.5 diabetes, but these diabetics must regain control of their intestinal brush border and liver by repairing leaky gut.

THE TYPE 2 DIABETES PROTOCOL

This protocol curative for type 2 diabetes is as follows:

1. Eat a ketogenic Paleolithic diet until your fasting blood glucose is constantly below 88. In my view, there are no safe starches for a diabetic until you regain your control of your fasting blood sugar. The ability to eat some starches, however, possibly may be recovered once fasting blood glucose is consistently below 88.

2. You must employ cold thermogenesis to shred your visceral fat. Instructions can be found online at: jackkruse.com/the-evolution-of-the-leptin-rx/

3. Coconut oil, ghee, and pastured butter should be your main sources of fuel in this plan.

4. Coconut oil has many benefits, including healing a leaky gut, which affects most diabetics. You can go back and read the VAP section in the chapter on labs to refresh yourself.

5. Coconut oil is antibacterial, antiviral, antifungal, and antiprotozoal. This means it stops infections to which diabetics are prone.

6. All diabetics should consider supplementation if they have certain complications, such as peripheral neuropathy. A recent study from the University of Utah showed that peripheral nerve damage occurs when blood sugar rises over 140 mg/dl (7.8 mmol/L) after meals. Most diabetics have low intracellular magnesium levels. Physicians test for serum magnesium, which is never accurate. You should consider getting the intracellular red blood cell magnesium test, called the "EXA Test" to assess your levels, as most diabetes are very deficient. If you are bad off, consider using epsom salt baths or foot soaks three times a week until the test improves, or use magnesium malate, aspartate, or citrate orally, from 800 to 1,600 mgs a day in divided doses. Its better to take it later at night because it helps sleep, too. It may cause some diarrhea, but that is not a big problem as you adjust with time.

7. I am a huge fan of vitamin D3 supplements daily and your target range is 60-100 ng/mL all year long. Do not use D2! This is conventional wisdom. We do not get vitamin D once a week or from D2, so why in the hell would you think this is how you should get it at the doctor's office. Replace it the way evolution designed is my advice.

8. I also heavily advocate vitamin K2 because of its effect on insulin resistance and your bone health, which was covered in the osteoporosis chapter.

9. I also think you need to consider hormone optimization to get back to optimal quicker. This includes all your hormones and not just the thyroid! Make sure to have your TPO antibodies and TGB antibodies checked to screen for autoimmune thyroid disease. Most cases of hypothyroidism in the United States are caused by Hashimoto's, an autoimmune disease that attacks and destroys the thyroid gland. Also, the higher your HS-CRP, is the longer it will take for leptin to regain control of all your hormones, so you may need to help your pituitary gland out.

10. What should you measure? I like tracking blood glucose, blood pressure, and sitting and standing heart rate every day for the first year. This will tell us when you regain leptin sensitivity and control of your sympathetic nervous system. I also suggest checking your cholesterol levels, mainly to monitor the triglyceride and HDL ratio, as this measures insulin sensitivity. I strive for a ratio of 2:1 or less.

If you are taking insulin, evaluate your C-peptide levels immediately after consuming a regular Coke or similar liquid candy to measure intrinsic maximal insulin production and your current pancreatic burden. Please remember that insulin is made from a very long molecule that is sliced down just as it leaves the pancreatic beta cell. This test tells us when you are recovering your beta cell insulin production. One piece folds up to be insulin and the other one floats off as C-peptide. By measuring C-peptide, we can avoid lab errors that often confuse endogenously made and injected insulin. If a patient has a C-peptide even as high as three or four and they are motivated to follow the ketogenic Paleolithic diet, they can see amazing results in as little as 10 days. Most type 2 diabetics can typically move their blood sugars into the normal range without the use of any drugs at all!

11. If you have peripheral neuropathy and severe fatty liver, you need to consider the use of whole body cold thermogenesis. It is yet unproven, but

I have a very interesting story about the mechanism of action and my own experience with it, explained in the last chapter of this book.

12. The reason we get diabetes is because somewhere in our evolutionary history, developing type 2 diabetes was advantageous. This is why I do not consider diabetes a true disease, but instead a symptom of a larger disorder. If it were not advantageous, we would have built-in systems to counterbalance it, which would have made itself evident by now. But there is a strong evolutionary reason we are prone to this disease, and the answer may surprise you. This was briefly covered in a book called Survival of the Sickest by Sharon Moalem, but did not hit the real gold of why I think evolution selected for diabetes. It is also explained in the last chapter of this book. This is why I look at type 2 diabetes as a symptom and not a straightforward Neolithic disease. The manner in which it has exploded in the 20th and 21st centuries is quite clear. It is a Neolithic disease caused by a biological mismatch created by man. There is too much evidence of multiple paths to this disease, and we see a huge variety of diabetics clinically. The best treatment, however, for most of those paths remains the Paleolithic diet.

YOU ARE EPI-PALEO NOW!

Why you need to look at your diabetic drugs and physician's recommendations differently today

When you have time, look at the The Action to Control Cardiovascular Risk in Diabetes (ACCORD) trial on the Internet. In it you will see disturbing findings of which most physicians are unaware. The ACCORD data showed that type 2 diabetics' lives are cut short by six years. This also held true in the treatment group, who had higher mortality rates despite lower HbA1c level and better blood glucoses with pharmaceutical use. It means all the crap you're taking is actually killing you and not really helping at all. It means that you must never become a diabetic, and if you do, you must eradicate the disease, not just treat your blood glucose with pharmaceuticals until you glycate yourself to death. The study showed that even with the best medical treatment and best drugs, you will have a shortened life. Why? Your mitochondria are not working well and are leaking energy. This ties directly to the length of telomeres, DNA sequences at the end of each chromosome that determine how long a cell can live. Diabetics have shorter telomeres because they age faster and their mitochondria are more leaky to free radicals. In essence, you "rust faster" and you don't have enough DW40 to bail you out, so you die sooner. If you want to live longer, eat a ketogenic Paleolithic diet.

Here is a link to a study by Lynda Frassetto, M.D. about the Paleolithic diet and diabetes. Read it and save your own life from conventional-wisdom advice.

Frassetto LA, Morris RC, Jr, Sebastian A. Metabolic and physiologic improvements from consuming a paleolithic, hunter-gatherer type diet. EJCN 63(8):947-55, 2009

If you change your diet you can lengthen your life and reverse type 2 diabetes. Moreover, type 1.5 diabetics who have had their beta cells fried by a leaky gut can reverse it often, too. No everyone with autoimmune diabetes can, but it certainly cannot hurt to try. People who are type 1 diabetics will need insulin, but even they will experience amazing results on the ketogenic version of the Paleolithic diet with time and patience. If one limits the inflammation of the plasma, all the secondary Neolithic diseases associated with diabetes fade-hypertension, sleep apnea, colon cancer, breast cancer, Alzheimer's disease, end-stage kidney disease, heart disease, and obesity. Paleolithic dieting improves mitochondrial energy production and life in general. But you must get this message loud and clear even if your physician does not, because you control what you buy and eat. All it requires is one new thought that may change your life.

REFERENCES

1. The Genetic Basis of Type 2 Diabetes Mellitus: Impaired Insulin Secretion versus Impaired Insulin Sensitivity. John E. Gerich. Endocrine Reviews 19(4) 491-503, 1998.
2. Hultberg M. Cysteine turnover in human cell lines is influenced by glyphosate (2007) Environmental Toxicology and Pharmacology, 24 (1), pp. 19-22
3. http://www.ncbi.nlm.nih.gov/pubmed/18719881
4. Clinical Risk Factors, DNA Variants, and the Development of Type 2 Diabetes Valeriya Lyssenko, M.D. et. al. New England Journal of Medicine, Volume 359:2220-2232, November 20, 2008,Number 21.
5. The T allele of rs7903146 TCF7L2 is associated with impaired insulinotropic action of incretin hormones, reduced 24 h profiles of plasma insulin and glucagon, and increased hepatic glucose production in young healthy men. K. Pilgaard et al. Diabetologia, Issue Volume 52, Number 7 / July, 2009. DOI 10.1007/s00125-009-1307-x

6. Stable Patterns of Gene Expression Regulating Carbohydrate Metabolism Determined by Geographic AncestryJonathan C. Schisler et. al. PLoS One 4(12): e8183. doi:10.1371/journal.pone.0008183

7. A variant near MTNR1B is associated with increased fasting plasma glucose levels and type 2 diabetes risk. Nabila Bouatia-Naji et al. Nature Genetics Published online: 7 December 2008, doi:10.1038/ng.277

8. http://www.sciencedaily.com/releases/2008/12/081207133817.htm

9. Glucose tolerance in adults after prenatal exposure to famine. Ravelli AC et al.Lancet. 1998 Jan 17;351(9097):173-7.,

10. Evidence of a Relationship Between Infant Birth Weight and Later Diabetes and Impaired Glucose Regulation in a Chinese Population Xinhua Xiao et. al. Diabetes Care31:483-487, 2008.

11. High Prevalence of Type 2 Diabetes and Pre-Diabetes in Adult Offspring of Women With Gestational Diabetes Mellitus or Type 1 Diabetes The role of intrauterine hyperglycemia Tine D. Clausen, MD et al. Diabetes Care 31:340-346, 2008

12. Diabetes in Relation to Serum Levels of Polychlorinated Biphenyls and Chlorinated Pesticides in Adult Native Americans Neculai Codru, Maria J. Schymura,Serban Negoita,Robert Rej,and David O. Carpenter.Environ Health Perspect. 2007 October; 115(10): 1442-1447.Published online 2007 July 17. doi: 10.1289/ehp.10315.

13. Intrauterine Exposure to Environmental Pollutants and Body Mass Index during the First 3 Years of Life Stijn L. Verhulst et al., Environmental Health Perspectives. Volume 117, Number 1, January 2009

14. Chronic Exposure to the Herbicide, Atrazine, Causes Mitochondrial Dysfunction and Insulin Resistance PLoS ONE Published 13 Apr 2009

15. http://www.sciencedaily.com/releases/2009/10/091009120846.htm

16. http://www.sciencedaily.com/releases/2007/08/070820175426.htm

17. http://www.sciencedaily.com/releases/2009/10/091009120846.htm

18. Arsenic Exposure and Prevalence of Type 2 Diabetes in US Adults. Ana Navas-Acien et al. JAMA. 2008;300(7):814-822.

19. Scott B. Patten et al. Psychother Psychosom 2009;78:182-186 (DOI: 10.1159/000209349)

20. Insulin resistance in the first-degree relatives of persons with Type 2 Diabetes. Straczkowski M et al. Med Sci Monit. 2003 May;9(5):CR186-90.

21. Beta cell (dys)function in non-diabetic offspring of diabetic patients M. Stadler et al. Diabetologia Volume 52, Number 11 / November, 2009, pp 2435-2444. doi 10.1007/s00125-009-1520-7

22. Impaired mitochondrial activity in the insulin-resistant offspring of patients with type 2 diabetes. Petersen KF et al. New England J Med 2004 Feb 12; 350(7);639-41

23. The role of skeletal muscle insulin resistance in the pathogenesis of the metabolic syndrome Petersen,KF et al. PNAS July 31, 2007 vol. 104 no. 31 12587-12594.

24. Downregulation of Diacylglycerol Kinase Delta Contributes to Hyperglycemia-Induced Insulin Resistance. Alexander V. Chibalin et. al. Cell, Volume 132, Issue 3, 375-386, 8 February 2008.

25. An isoenergetic very low carbohydrate diet improves serum HDL cholesterol and triacylglycerol concentrations, the total cholesterol to HDL cholesterol ratio and postprandial lipemic responses compared with a low fat diet in normal weight, normolipidemic women. Volek JS, et al. J Nutr. 2003 Sep;133(9):2756-61.

26. Very low-carbohydrate and low-fat diets affect fasting lipids and postprandial lipemia differently in overweight men. Sharman MJ, et al. J Nutr. 2004 Apr;134(4):880-5.

27. http://mend.endojournals.org/content/16/7/1612.full.pdf

28. http://www.jbc.org/content/272/44/27758.full.pdf

29. http://www.jbc.org/content/273/47/31160.short

30. Increased prevalence of impaired glucose tolerance in patients with painful sensory neuropathy. Singleton, JR Smith AG, Bromberg, MB Diabetes Care 24 (8) 1448-1453 2001.

31. Value of the Oral Glucose Tolerance Test in the Evaluation of Chronic Idiopathic Axonal Polyneuropathy. Charlene Hoffman-Snyder; Benn E. Smith; Mark A. Ross; Jose Hernandez; E. Peter Bosch. Arch Neurol. 2006;63:1075-1079.

32. The spectrum of neuropathy in diabetes and impaired glucose tolerance. C.J. Sumner, MD, S. Sheth, MBBS MPH, J.W. Griffin, MD, D.R. Cornblath, MD and M. Polydefkis, MD; Neurology 2003;60:108-111.

33. Prevalence of Polyneuropathy in Pre-Diabetes and Diabetes Is Associated With Abdominal Obesity and Macroangiopathy Dan Ziegler et al. Diabetes Care 31:464-469, 2008

34. Krinsley, James, Effect of an Intensive Glucose Management Protocol on the Mortality of Critically Ill Adult Patients. Mayo Clinic Proc. Jan 2004, p. 992-1000.

35. Relation between fasting glucose and retinopathy for diagnosis of diabetes: three population-based cross-sectional studies Wong TY, et al Lancet 2008; 371: 736-743.

36. Astiz M., Alaniz M.J.T.d, Marra C.A. Effect of pesticides on cell survival in liver and brain rat tissues (2009) Ecotoxicology and Environmental Safety, 72 (7), pp. 2025-2032.

37. Culver AL, et al. Statin Use and Risk of Diabetes Mellitus in Postmenopausal Women in the Women's Health Initiative. Arch Intern Med. 2012;0(2012):20116252-9.

38. Walter Arnold, Thomas Ruf, Fredy Frey-Roos, Ute Bruns.Diet-Independent Remodeling of Cellular Membranes Precedes Seasonally Changing Body Temperature in a Hibernator. PLoS ONE, 2011; 6 (4): e18641 DOI:10.1371/journal.pone.00186412.

39. http://www.sciencedaily.com/releases/2012/02/120215123352.htm

40. http://www.sciencedaily.com/releases/2011/04/110413171323.htm?utm_source=feedburner&utm_medium=feed&utm_campaign=Feed%3A+sciencedaily+%28ScienceDaily%3A+Latest+Science+News%293

Chapter Nine

HEART DISEASE AND THE EPI-PALEO RX

CONVENTIONAL WISDOM HEART DISEASE RX:

According to conventional wisdom, eating saturated fat elevates cholesterol, putting you at risk for a heart attack. The lipid hypotheses put forth by Rudolf Virchow in 1856 says that blood lipid (fat) accumulation in arterial walls causes atherosclerosis and heart disease. The diet-heart hypothesis says that saturated fat and dietary cholesterol elevate cholesterol and lipids in our blood, which causes heart disease and atherosclerosis. These two hypotheses are often mixed up but they both form the foundation of conventional dogma in medicine today.

Other conventional risk factors for cardiovascular disease include high concentrations of low-density lipoprotein (LDL), low concentrations of high-density lipoprotein (HDL), diabetes, a history of smoking, and a family history of heart disease. Other factors that may influence the progression of heart disease include C-reactive protein (CRP, an inflammatory marker), and fibrinogen (a pro-coagulant marker).

Patients with a heart disease risk of less than 10 percent over 10 years are considered to be "low risk." Added risk factors of CRP and homocysteine go above and beyond conventional risk factors and conventional cardiology does not use them as a screening tool.

If you fall into a low-risk category they do not recommend you consider advanced testing, such as high-sensitivity CRP (HS-CRP), homocysteine, ECG, ETT, and EBTC. In their view, ECG, ETT, and EBCT have poor accuracy for predicting coronary heart disease (CHD) events among asymptomatic adults.

This, of course, assumes they know what the underlying cause of heart disease really is. That is for you to decide after looking at this from an evolutionary medicine perspective, as their view is based on conventional allopathic wisdom.

This next comment comes directly from the government's website discussing cardiac health disease screening. It says, "Screening tests for CHD should not be routinely offered to asymptomatic, low risk adults. They should only be offered on a case-by-case basis to patients at increased risk when you judge that the benefits to the individual patient outweigh the harms. Patients may ask about getting screened with these tests as a result of community health fairs, direct-to-consumer advertising, or health experiences of a friend or family member. Consider the patient's request respectfully. Discuss the patient's concerns and provide more information if needed."

Here is the link to the page I pulled this from: http://www.prevention.va.gov/Screening_for_Coronary_Heart_Disease.asp#riskdetermined

It appears the government does not want you screened if you don't meet their risk criteria. But what if they are looking for the wrong things? Might you be at risk and not know it with these guidelines? If you don't look for something, it is often hard to find.

HERE IS HOW THEY SUGGEST WE TREAT HEART DISEASE:

1. Offer help to quit smoking. Primal Rx suggests this, too. We are in complete agreement!

2. Increase physical activity. Primal Rx asks, "How do I best do this?" They send you to a cardiac rehab specialist who tells you to do a lot of cardio exercise along with your low-fat, high-carbohydrate diet filled with "heart-healthy" whole grains.

3. Maintain a healthy weight. Primal Rx asks, "How do I best do this?" They send you to a nutritionist or dietician whose curriculum was funded by the USDA and who advocates grains for health.

4. Regularly screen for hypertension and high cholesterol. Primal Rx asks, "Why should I have to do this if I eat correctly?" Lab companies love this recommendation, but no one likes it better than big pharma. You will be asked to take drugs that don't help you prevent death, and may, in fact, make you very ill while making you broke.

5. Control diabetes, hypertension, and high cholesterol if present. Primal Rx asks, "Why do I have these disorders to begin with?" Because the American Heart Association diet causes hypertension.

6. Consider aspirin therapy for men with increased CHD risk. Primal Rx says, "Doesn't aspirin cause a leaky gut, which causes inflammation? Why would I want to do this?"

7. Work with patients to increase their motivation to change, help them set goals, and learn to problem-solve as needed. Primal Rx asks, "OK, how does your doctor do this? A prescription for a statin and a diet loaded with whole grains and low in red meat is what they tell us while giving us prescriptions for synthetic drugs every, and still millions die of heart disease. WOW!"

BRIEF OVERVIEW OF HEART DISEASE TODAY

Heart disease was the number-one disease affecting Americans in 2010. The World Health Organization's statistics showed 31.5 percent of women and 26.8 percent of men die of heart disease-it's the number-one killer of men and women in the United States, and has been since the early 1900s. Each year the prevalence grew, eventually catching Washington's attention. It reached a frenzy when Dwight Eisenhower had three heart attacks and then died from a massive heart attack. Did you know that when he died his cholesterol was below 150?

In the 1940s, the U.S. government became interested in cardiovascular disease and began the Framingham Heart study. To date this is the best study on cardiovascular disease we have in human history. This study spanned the years 1948-1998. However, what the study found and what many panels of experts said it found are not congruent. As a result, the public to this day thinks high cholesterol causes heart disease, a belief that has dictated how the National Institutes of Health and the federal government have spent close to $60 billion researching treatment and a cure. Neither goal has been reached. In the United States, we have used medical journals, organized medicine and all its specialties, medical school curriculums, dietitian curriculums, and nutritionist curriculums to teach the belief that elevated total cholesterol is the ultimate cause of cardiovascular disease and heart attacks, heart failure, and eventually death. I will explain the reality of this uncontrolled experiment on 300,000 million people during the last 50 years in our country.

People who follow a low-fat, high-carbohydrate diet and take statins to lower their cholesterol still succumb to heart disease as the number-one cause of death! The results are woeful. And yet we have cardiology telling us that heart disease is falling. Yes, if you use mirrors and tricks of statistics. I let overall mortality guide my thinking. If people still are dying from heart disease more than any other cause, it means we do not know how to treat it.

If people follow conventional advice and still die from heart disease, maybe the question is wrong. Maybe fats have nothing to do with heart disease. Neither of which is being considered, by the way. No one can fathom that lipids might not be the cause, because we have 50 years of data saying they are. Instead, their focus is on newer generation drugs to lower LDL cholesterol even further.

In my medical career, I have seen the recommended LDL levels for humans plummet based upon no good science. We have been recommending against saturated fats and cholesterol levels for the last 80 years, but heart disease remains the number-one killer of men and women. The reality is that saturated fats and dietary cholesterol likely are preventative to heart disease! Yes, you heard that correctly. Heart disease is caused by cellular inflammation that begins in the gastrointestinal tract and is heavily influenced by our hormonal response. Chris Masterjohn, a PhD candidate at the University of Connecticut gave an excellent talk at the Ancestral Health Symposium in August of 2011, describing heart disease as a disease that "involves molecular degeneration and cellular miscommunication."

Time and time again in studies on heart disease risk, the best measure of cardiovascular risk is the HDL level. The National Heart Foundation of New Zealand published an absolute risk calculator that uses a ratio of total cholesterol to HDL, a much better predictor of coronary artery disease risk than is the total cholesterol alone.

It seems in New Zealand they get this, but here in the United States your doctor is trying to lower your LDL cholesterol to ensure you get cancer! The link of low LDL with cancer is well documented in the literature. When a cell divides, it uses something called a "mitotic spindle" to line up our 46 chromosomes so they can split into 23 in each offspring cell. The mitotic spindle is made from cholesterol. When your LDL cholesterol goes below 200, we begin to see defects in the formation of this spindle, causing uneven chromosomal separation called "aneuploidy." Aneuploidy is a precursor to cancer. Ask your oncologist if this is true, or Google it. This is why more than 15 major trials on cholesterol show a link between low LDL cholesterol and cancer risk.

WHAT DOES A LOW HDL REALLY MEAN IN TERMS OF HORMONES?

Low HDL predicts a high cardiovascular risk in one's lifetime. Low HDL walks hand-in-hand with high inflammation. This is best measured by HS-CRP. I fully expect HS-CRP to be usurped by assays that directly measure inflammatory cytokines. These tests are currently available by many labs but are not covered by insurance, so few people even know about them. They are more accurate and sensitive than an HS-CRP. Is a cytokine panel a great test for heart disease risk? Not by itself, but right now the best way to assess your real risk of cardiovascular disease is to use an array of tests. HDL is one, and a leaky gut is the first thing to look at when HDL is low. We covered this extensively in the lipid profile section in the chapter on testing. HS-CRP, homocysteine, EKG findings, cytokine array sampling, lower IGF-1 levels, coronary calcium index scans, and a triglyceride to HDL ratio (below 2:1) are other good ones for you to assess yourself.

The real story behind cholesterol and heart disease is found in oxidized cholesterol. Cholesterol levels do not matter. However, how long our cholesterol is exposed to our plasma is important if our plasma is oxidized. Inflammation directly oxidizes our plasma. This means that heart disease prevention should be focused on inflammation, not cholesterol.

This is the low-density cholesterol that is left to circulate in our blood too long, becoming oxidized and raising the risk for atherosclerosis formation in major arteries. What causes low-density particles to stay in the blood's circulation too long? There are many. A poor functioning LDL receptor, low T3 levels, poor functioning cholesterol ester transfer protein (CETP) enzyme, and low sex-steroid hormones are big cardiac risk factors. If you have a chronically elevated HS-CRP, you generally are in deep trouble. This tends to walk hand-in-hand with a low Vitamin D level, too.

HORMONES AND HEART DISEASE

The major hormones are linked to heart disease: low testosterone, low estrogen, low thyroid hormones, and low vitamin D. Remember, leptin resistance is seen with all of these hormonal abnormalities. The final nail in the coffin is that chronically elevated cortisol is also seen with leptin resistance and heart disease. So it appears that every hormonal disruption correlated with leptin resistance is also seen in cardiovascular disease. This means a person who is leptin resistant is also at severe risk for heart disease. Even conventional medicine does not screw this correlation up. But they fail to realize that leptin resistance is the real source of the problem.

Leptin controls all the other hormones in our body. When we are leptin resistant we can expect low T3, low testosterone, low estrogen, and low vitamin D levels. Let me ask you this, when have you ever heard of a cardiologist looking at your hormone panel to assess heart disease risk? I thought so. They look at your lipid panel as their only proxy, when they should also consider HS-CRP, homocysteine, and a hormone panel. They should also look in an area where there is an easy assessment to make-the oral cavity. If you have periodontal disease (loose teeth with bleeding gums) you have inflammation that can cause your heart a problem. If you have a lot of tartar on your teeth that becomes easily calcified you have a Vitamin K2 deficiency, which the Framingham Heart study also linked to heart disease risk. A lack of Vitamin K2 is tied to another hormone problem that most do not know about, the hormone osteocalcin. Do you suffer from a lot of sore throats and canker sores in your mouth? The same family of bacteria that is involved in the development of dental caries also is related to the development of canker sores and to an increased risk of cardiovascular disease. This is how you make connections to risks without fancy testing. You can look in your own mouth for bleeding during brushing or flossing. You can ask your dentist if your dental tartar is calcified or not. I have several blogs on my website about the links between oral health and overall health. Heart disease risk is associated with changes we can easily monitor in our own mouths.

THE HORMONE CASCADE AND HEART DISEASE RISK

Now we need to examine why each hormone is tied to cardiovascular disease risk. T3, the active form of thyroid hormone, and vitamin A are required for the conversion of LDL cholesterol to pregnenolone, which is the precursor of all steroid hormones in humans. So if T3 is low, you cannot convert excess cholesterol made in response to acute stress to make the correct hormones. This is why thyroid disease is linked to cardiovascular disease in just about every human study done on cardiovascular disease.

Thyroid hormone binds to its receptor and activates the thyroid response element (TRE). This binding immediately alters the cell's gene expression to facilitate production of LDL receptors. The LDL receptors then clear the plasma of small, dense LDL and oxidized LDL, which are like "landfills of toxins" in our blood. So sufficient thyroid hormone activity is necessary for this process to work.

As humans age, pregnenolone is the first hormone that usually falls off a cliff. This happens most commonly around 40-45 years old. If you see this, it tells you that your cells are not making enough of this critical building block from LDL cholesterol. Often times this is because a protein called "sterol regulatory element (SRE)," which is required for cholesterol synthesis and uptake, is affected by inflammation caused by excessive polyunsaturated fatty acid (PUFA) accumulation as we age. This is often why eating dietary cholesterol has little effect on serum lipid levels. Instead, high omega-6 levels may starve our cells of cholesterol needed to make hormones. Again, here we have the Rosetta Stone of our hormone levels to give us insight into the health of our coronary vessels. High PUFAs can also provide a link between heart disease, peripheral artery disease, and the development of Alzheimer's disease in the brain.

Here is another interesting point most physicians seem to have forgotten. In response to acute stress from trauma, burns, infections, emotional trauma, or excess exercise, the human liver RAISES cholesterol production to allow for REPAIR. Evolution designed our bodies to raise our cholesterol in response to stress! We do this by activating the SRE I mentioned earlier. This is but another reason to stop buying the belief that cholesterol is inherently sinister to our longevity. Cholesterol is actually a "bandaid for damage" in normal cellular physiology, and it is an antioxidant too! So how did it get its sinister reputation? Sloppy research and intellectual laziness thrown together with "experts" working for the pharmaceutical companies making cholesterol-lowering drugs is the answer. I hope you read Anthony Colpo's book, The Great Cholesterol Con. Anthony is a trip if you read his blog, but this gentlemen wrote a brilliant treatise on why you need to call BS on every dogmatic belief organized medicine has about heart disease. When you read it, you will become sick to your stomach. I know I did. I don't enjoy being lied to either.

WHERE DOES HOMOCYSTEINE FIT IN CARDIOVASCULAR RISK ASSESSMENTS?

Homocysteine is a byproduct of methionine, one of the building blocks of protein. This breakdown cannot be completed nor reversed when there is a deficiency of one of four substances-vitamins B6, folic acid, vitamin B12, and betaine, a nutrient important for heart and blood vessel function. Homocysteine has a similar history to cholesterol. Families with very high levels of homocysteine due to genetic mutations show a very increased risk of cardiovascular disease, and high levels are also associated with 10 percent of the risk variance among middle-aged males. Cholesterol accounts for a smaller proportion. Correcting the appropriate deficiency often relieves symptoms of high homocysteine, such as fatigue, balance problems, and sleep disturbances. It is definitely not a case of "pie in the sky."

However, the most recent Cochrane review on the subject concluded that there is no evidence that reducing homocysteine with vitamins will reduce the risk of cardiovascular disease. Many thought this review would put to bed the homocysteine issue, but after reviewing this more closely and reading their statements, I cannot advocate that position. For example, they stated, "It is interesting to mention the HOPE-2 2006 study (which showed a significant reduction of stroke) was the only study to use an adequate dose of vitamin B12." Well, that is a huge factor that could skew the data badly. It appears none of the studies looked at whether patients had an H. pylori infection, which causes vitamin B12 and folate deficiency. It is also a significant cause of leaky gut, which can lead to oxidized plasma, and directly affect LDL receptor activity in the liver, all of which raise cardiovascular risk. It also appeared in the studies that none of them used injections of vitamin B12. They likely used oral concoctions, which clearly are not as good as the injectable forms when one suffers from a leaky gut and poor nutrient absorption. I think the jury should still be out, and this is why I still look at homocysteine, even on myself. It has been one of the rare times I do not think the Cochrane review is rigorous enough.

On my website I have written about why we need to pay attention to the B vitamins because they are tied to energy metabolism in many pathways. B vitamins are critical to how these pathways interact with one another for optimal function. A primal bio-hacker would do well to pay attention to optimal B levels. If you eat well you may not have to worry about them. But that is assuming you are absorbing everything you eat, and if you have a leaky gut that is a bad assumption. We are only what we absorb, not what we see ourselves eating. Many people waste their money on great primal food because they do not repair their gut lining first. This is critical in heart disease, autoimmune diseases, inflammatory bowel diseases, depression, and autism spectrum disorders.

A FINAL WORD ABOUT STATINS

If you have any doubt statins are worthless, you might want to read the scathing review by Michel de Lorgeril, MD in the Annals of Internal Medicine recently published. After this was published, I thought that most doctors would stop writing about statins for primary prevention of heart disease. I knew the cardiologists would not stop because they all are married to their specialty's dogma, which is tied directly to the lipid hypothesis.

You need to know about the Jupiter trial (Justification for the Use of Statins in Primary Prevention: An Intervention Trial Evaluating Rosuvastatin). This trial and De Lorgeril's response was reviewed in an excellent blog named Diets and Science on January 9, 2012, and I want to share it with you here because it is vital information for those on a statin today:

"Dr. de Lorgeril notes that the results of cholesterol-lowering drug trials show no evidence that statin drugs lower the disease rates or death rates of people with or without coronary heart disease with one exception, and that is the JUPITER (Justification for the Use of Statins in Primary Prevention) trial. JUPITER reports a substantial decrease in the risk of cardiovascular diseases among patients without coronary heart disease and with normal or low cholesterol levels.

The results of the JUPITER study were met with a massive media fanfare proclaiming the benefits of statin drugs. This enthusiastic recommendation has no doubt persuaded many people with normal cholesterol levels to start long term statin treatment.

The JUPITER trial tested the effects of rosuvastatin (Crestor) in patients without heart disease and with normal or low cholesterol levels but relatively high levels of C-reactive protein, a marker of inflammation. The study spanned 1,315 sites in 26 countries and included 17,802 people who were assigned either 20 mg/d of rosuvastatin or placebo.

Three recent trials with rosuvastatin (with the acronyms CORONA, GISSI-HF and AURORA) had been conducted, and all had failed to provide evidence that rosuvastatin therapy reduces heart disease complications at all.

The JUPITER trial was prematurely terminated on the grounds that it had generated evidence that the statin treatment had definitely reduced heart disease rates.

However the evidence shows otherwise:

(a) If you include people who had fatal and nonfatal heart attack and stroke-the trial was stopped after only 240 incidents.

(b) There was no difference in the incidence of serious adverse events (total hospitalizations, prolongations of hospitalizations, cancer, and permanent disability) between the 2 groups.

(c) There was hardly any difference in death rates when the trial was ended, and the trend was showing that the statin groups death rate was increasing compared to the placebo group.

An 'unequivocal reduction in cardiovascular mortality' was announced in March 2008 as the main justification for the premature trial termination.

However the actual facts again beg to differ:

(d) Fatal heart attacks were 9 in the statin group and 6 in the placebo group.

(e) Stroke death was 3 in the statin group compared to 6 taking the placebo.

So there was 12 cardiovascular deaths in each group. Hardly an 'unequivocal reduction in cardiovascular mortality' as the JUPITER study authors concluded.

So why was the trial really stopped early? You will not like this part at all!

As stated earlier JUPITER was hailed in the media as a ringing endorsement for us all to start statin therapy. This was achieved by the authors of the study only highlighting some results of the trial and completely ignoring other, less favorable data. It also raises the suspicion that if the trial had continued then the results would have shown statins in an even more unfavorable light.

Rosuvastatin (sold under the brand name Crestor) is marketed and distributed by AstraZeneca Pharmaceuticals.

The JUPITER trial involved multiple conflicts of interest:

(f) It was conducted by Astra Zeneca with their obvious commercial interests.

(g) Nine of 14 authors of the JUPITER article have financial ties to the Astra Zeneca.

(h) The principal investigator has a personal conflict of interest as a co-holder of the patent for the C-reactive protein test.

(i) Astra Zeneca's own investigators controlled and managed the raw data, which increases the chance of bias appearing in the data.

Dr. de Lorgeril concluded:

1. The results of the JUPITER trial are clinically inconsistent and therefore should not influence medical practice or clinical guidelines.

2. The results of the JUPITER trial show that commercially sponsored clinical trials are at risk of poor quality and bias.

3. The failure of the JUPITER trial to demonstrate a protective effect of rosuvastatin confirms the results of more than 12 other cholesterol-lowering trials published in recent years, which all provided no evidence of protection against heart disease by cholesterol lowering. (Dr. De Lorgeril is a great doctor in my opinion for saying it loud in the literature)

4. These failed trials strongly suggest that the presumed preventive effects of cholesterol-lowering drugs have been considerably exaggerated.

Dr. de Lorgeril ends by saying that the time has come for a critical reappraisal of ALL cholesterol-lowering and statin treatments for the prevention of heart disease, and the emphasis on pharmaceuticals for the prevention of heart disease has diverted individual and public health attention away from other proven methods of prevention such as a healthy lifestyle, exercise and diet."

◇◇

The FDA just released a warning label for statins. This is the first sign of incremental changes that must happen. In my medical opinion, statins are not fit for human consumption. Their mechanism of action blocks hormone production, alters cellular signaling, and blocks formation of mitotic spindles. These actions cause widespread metabolic problems that affect cognition, cause muscle and back pain, lower hormone responses, worsen diabetes, and create a strong link to cancer because of their effect on chromosomal cleavage. None of these side effects is worth the benefit based upon the current research on these drugs. Moreover, I do not believe LDL cholesterol has much to do with heart disease. I think it has more do to with the length of time LDL cholesterol is bathing in oxidized plasma. These things can be controlled with an anti-inflammatory diet and the cold thermogenesis protocol listed on my website.

My advice is if you want to be optimal, dump every statin you're on ASAP. When your physician hands you a prescription for them, be kind, put it in your pocket, and save the prescription folded up in the jacket of a Paleo book. After you use the Primal Rx to regain your health, you then should hand your doctor a copy of your Paleo book with the folded prescriptions in them and say, "Doc, I think you need this book more than I do now." That action will move some physicians to think and maybe even transform. Physicians are good people stuck in a bad system. You must remember physician reimbursement is tied to writing that statin prescription. This is another reason the healthcare system must be transformed. It is set up to keep you sick. Hospitals need illness and disease to stay afloat. In the new system I envision, doctors can return to keeping people well, and hospitals can shrink in numbers and size, be centralized, and controlled by the government. We would rely less on them as a population if we employ the Primal Rx, as our need for major procedures would fall off tremendously. We will always need hospitals for some medical issues, such as trauma and disaster response, but in my opinion this is a system that should be ideally controlled by government to allow for a standard of access for emergencies.

THE PRIMAL RX FOR HEART DISEASE PREVENTION

1. Use every test you want to monitor your cardiac risk. You should not limit testing, as the government or cardiologists say, because the data is still not clear as to what is the major cause of heart disease. This includes IGF-1 levels in heart disease. We need to optimize our vitamin D levels as laid out in the chapter on labs. Vitamin D optimization is among the cheapest and easiest hacks we can do for our heart. I think as research continues, vitamin D will be shown to significantly mitigate cardiac risks while simultaneously driving the incidence of cardiac disease down. We can do this right now ourselves without much risk.

2. When it comes to LDL, the larger the particle size, the better off you are. That trend is clear. Eating carbs causes a pattern of small, dense LDL, which favors heart disease, and eating saturated fat and protein do not. I am not against particle size testing, but I think for the uninformed it can generate confusion. Sometimes, having more choices can limit our ability to make a decision. For this reason, I do not routinely recommend advanced particle size testing like William Davis, M.D. does in his online Track your Plaque program. I also fully believe that if you eat a primal template, you are guaranteeing that your particle size is large and fluffy. If you have leaky gut however, I see great utility in particle testing because the results may shed light on how good your ability to treat your own gut is. It is a measuring stick for your own treatment plan. What I think is clear, however, is that the level of oxidized cholesterol we have is the most significant risk factor for cardiovascular disease because of the time cholesterol may spend suspended in our oxidized plasma. If we improve LDL clearance and decrease the cytokines in our plasma, we essentially limit all our risks.

LDL oxidation, not concentration, determines the macrophage uptake of cholesterol in our liver. The future PhD holder, Chris Masterjohn, made this point brilliantly in his talk at the 2011 Ancestral Health Symposium. We need to heed it. Inflammation is the source for oxidized cholesterol, and the number-one portal for inflammation is our guts. It also appears inflammation is the number-one risk factor for atherosclerosis and peripheral artery disease, so we need to be mindful of this as well.

3. What is quite clear is that one must eat a primal template to lower the risk of cardiac disease. This is cornerstone principle. The primary reason this diet works is because it best supports the endogenous (internal) antioxidant system without supplements, and it optimizes our thyroid status while properly regulating the generation of inflammatory cascades. Let's dive into some science here. The Paleolithic diet is best known for advocating a low omega 6 level and a higher omega 3 level. By having an omega 6/3 ratio below 4/1, we suppress formation of PGE2 and leukotriene B4, which are both very inflammatory and destroy our hormonal responses. This is what alters our epigenetic switches. The SAD provides processed carbs and PUFAs that specifically raise this flame-throwing chemicals, driving up HS-CRP. But the Paleolithic diet lowers IL-6, TNF alpha, TNF beta, IL-1b, and IL-8, which are our first-line cytokine responses. Few test these cytokines, but each one causes very specific biochemical alterations that affect the pathways of how cells signal one another and the brain. (The most important cellular signals for us to test are the hormonal responses.) These cytokines are behind every Neolithic disease known to man. We do not test for these often because the testing is not covered by insurance and it costs a lot of money. I am hoping soon that we can abandon HS-CRP and use cytokine panels instead. They are way more sensitive and specific. We can make major predictions that are quite accurate when we know this information.

Conventional wisdom says saturated fats are a major cause of heart disease, but a very a recent meta-analysis does not favor this view. Instead, it supports a primal diet. The Harvard study, done in 2010 by Dariush Mozaffarian, M.D., showed that when the USDA recommends we replace saturated fats in our diet with carbs, heart disease is the result. The study was comprehensive and well done, and showed that replacing saturated fat with carbohydrates raised triglyceride levels and lowered HDL levels. It went further to show this dietary change did not raise or lower the ratio of total cholesterol to HDL, and suggested saturated fats play no role at all in heart disease. This data should have moved organized cardiology, or at least Dr. Oz., but it fell on deaf ears.

I suggest you use this information wisely if you have heart disease. I advocate plenty of saturated fat in my own diet. Coconut oil has been my number-one diesel fuel since 2007. Now, in 2012, I have proof that my Primal Sense was right all along. The Paleolithic diet provides for saturated fats, very low levels of PUFAs, low carbohydrate exposures, and limits most processed foods that stimulate inflammation. This is why it is a core element in the Primal Rx.

4. The omega 6/3 ratio: This is precisely why controlling your balance of omega 6 to 3 plays a leading role in keeping you healthy. It also supports intracellular signaling in the heart for optimal functioning. For the cardiac system, IL-6 is the most important cytokine. How did I come up with this? Well, I met a cardiologist at a meeting who told me that we know today that the human heart fails because of a breakdown of the cellular process called autophagy. Autophagy is the process cellular renewal that occurs while we sleep. He shared with me studies done at UCLA that showed that heart failure is directly tied to autographic failure. He also went on to explain that people with severe heart failure who could not meet the criteria for transplant surgery did extremely well with growth hormone. Growth hormone is released during two stages of our sleep and helps facilitate the process of autophagy. I already knew from my readings that growth hormone was important in sleep biology and muscle physiology. Autophagy is how the heart renews itself to function well. If you do not sleep well, you tend to have cardiac disease. This is why most people with sleep disorders have serious cardiac risk factors. Ernst von Schwarz, MD, PhD, a cardiologist at UCLA, will be the principal investigator of a prospective study on growth hormone use for adult humans. In my opinion, this study has been needed for years because conventional medicine has frowned on growth hormone. I have always thought this was shortsighted and needed a rigorous study for heart patients. If this works, it can save people from stenting and surgery and we need to consider it.

When I heard this a few years ago, I linked to an article I read in the 90s about how DHEA levels are very low in people with poor sleep. I searched the Internet and found that low DHEA levels are linked dramatically to high IL-6 levels, which causes inflammation. When I made this link I realized how to go after different diseases by monitoring hormonal responses as a guide. The SAD promotes high levels of IL-6, as does obesity. This is why diabetes, heart disease, and obesity all walk together. And this is also why these patients tend to sleep poorly. I then kept digging at every other disease I knew. I found links everywhere. Remember that IL-6 is very chemically similar to leptin. This link blew my mind. I then found every

Neolithic disease was tied to this inflammation and leptin at some level. I began writing all this down and trying to figure out which cytokine caused which hormone level to crater. It was a Rosetta Stone moment. I began to write my Quilt document to explain the interconnectedness of the system. This document can be found at my website. I also found some more data about heart disease, or lack there of, much later from another former dentist and a Paleoanthropologist.

That former dentist was Weston A. Price, who said it was quite rare of to see a cardiac death in the native peoples he studied during his travels. These are all covered in his masterpiece work, Nutrition and Physical Degeneration. The native Inuit exhibit this as well. I distinctly remember being a young boy on a field trip at the Museum of Natural History in New York City and learning that Dr. Albert Schweitzer was floored to find no evidence of cancer in the native Inuit. I now know this was no coincidence, it was evolutionary biology at work. Because they ate in manners congruent to their environment, heart disease did not seem to be present in many hunter gatherer groups worldwide. I also recently learned that the Mars Candy corporation found a camp of hunter gatherers in the Amazon jungle who have never had a person in their tribe suffer any coronary event. They do an unusual thing in their diet. They put ground chocolate in every bit of water they drink throughout their entire life. Chocolate is loaded with resveratrol and other polyphenols that destroy IL-6 and raise DHEA levels. The use of 99 percent, pure organic chocolate (low mycotoxin) is now part of my own Primal Rx for heart disease prevention because of these findings. The reason this works is that it activates part of the ancient leptin-melanocortin pathway that all mammals possess. This confers longevity and health when you live in this pathway chronically.

It does seem that the European chocolates, such as Lindt, have much lower levels of mycotoxins present in them. If you are going to use these to protect your heart, make sure that what you use is not offsetting the cardiac benefit with inflammation. Using a good quality chocolate is certainly cheaper than statins, and more effective, too.

In our country, we face tremendous risks for cardiac disease because we eat a man-made diet with many processed foods. Those people with higher cardiac risks should consider altering their diets to a ketogenic version of the primal diet, using mostly coconut oil for its high lauric acid and myristic acid content, and its huge benefits to cardiac metabolism. The heart actually prefers to burn palmitic oil, which is a saturated fat.

5. You need to do everything possible to increase your LDL receptor activity in your liver-this one maneuver abolishes most of the risks we see in cardiovascular disease. Remember, the liver is part of the gut, so the leaky gut Rx is critical here. Small amounts of alcohol elevate LDL receptor activity. I generally advocate Argentine Malbecs and French Pinot Noirs because both have the highest amounts of resveratrol. White wines with high levels of resveratrol are rieslings from Long Island, New York. Most California wines are grown using pesticides to diminish fungal growth, and these pesticides severely restrict the formation of resveratrol in the wine, so I am not a big fan of them. There are some organic producers I favor, but these wines are quite pricey because of increased production costs. One of those premium producers is Neal Vineyards on Howell Mountain in California's Napa Valley. With wine, you must remember the dose makes the poison. One glass of red wine every night is not a problem. One bottle of wine per night is a problem and you will see the effects in your lowered HDL levels and poor sleep at night if you drink to excess. I think 4 ounces for women and 6 ounces for men a day is fine for optimal health. This is not an Rx to become a booze-hound!

The other way to modulate your LDL receptor is to make sure your hormone levels are optimized, too! This includes your thyroid panels, your sex steroid levels, and your vitamin D levels. Lower pregnenolone, progesterone, and DHEA levels all correlate with heart disease. Elevated 24-hour total cortisol (salivary testing) and cortisol out of its normal diurnal rhythms also put you at risk for heart disease. If your normal diurnal rhythms are off this destroys sleep quality and quantity, reducing the process of autophagy in the heart. Remember, the number-one way the human heart fails is via autophagic failure, not apoptotic (programmed cell death) failure. Poor sleep is a major risk factor for heart disease from an evolutionary prism. This is why so many people with sleep apnea die of right-sided heart failure. It is also why we find that heart attacks and deaths have a striking diurnal pattern of when they occur in humans in many studies.

6. High-intensity weight training is among the best way to get your LDL receptor back to optimal while simultaneously raising your HDL.

Look to experts such as Greg Everett (caathletics.com), Mark Rippetoe (startingstrength.com), and the massive contribution of research by Frank Booth, PhD. They advocate the correct forms and ways to exercise. Exercise increases HDL while increasing testosterone and growth hormone secretion, which are both cardio-protective and support muscle growth. This includes our heart muscles. There is now new data to support the use of growth hormone for patients with terminal heart failure. If it works for a completely failed heart, you know it must perform wonders in your own heart as you exercise your way to naturally high growth hormone levels! You can follow growth hormone levels to see how your exercise program is working for you. My growth hormone went up close to 100 percent in my first year of full exercise, without any drugs. This is a pretty constant feature in most humans.

7. Mindfulness is a key part of the Primal Rx for heart disease. This has been shown in many "blue zone studies" of places where people live long lives. It is one of the better ways to lower cortisol and stress. Lower cortisol levels have been associated with lower cardiac risk across the board in the literature. An abnormal diurnal pattern of cortisol, however, I believe has a much greater effect than total cortisol on heart disease propagation in humans. I believe this is because of the effects on sleep. Having high evening levels of cortisol and low morning cortisol levels should be aggressively treated.

8. A word about the APoE4 allele, the genetic marker for Alzheimer's, and the Primal Rx. Fifteen to 20 percent of the world's population seem to be APoE4 carriers, meaning they have one copy of the gene. Only 2 percent of the world has both copies. Having this gene supposedly puts the carrier at an elevated risk for heart disease and Alzheimer's disease. If you have high total cholesterol and high small, dense LDL cholesterol while eating a primal template, what should you do? According to genetic linkage studies, people from Scotland and Scandinavia appear to have the highest risk for carrying this allele. An interesting evolutionary theory is that this occurred because the ApoE4 allele allowed humans to tolerate lower vitamin D from the decreasing amount of sunlight as they migrated from the tropics toward the poles. Grace Cathome (of drbganimalpharm.blogspot.com) wrote a fabulous blog piece about this issue in which she

correctly stated, "the density of the lipoproteins (LDL) determines its function. Small, dense LDL is damaging because it is most susceptible to oxidation in our plasma. For ApoE4 patients, dietary carbohydrates and dietary deficiencies of saturated fat dramatically shape and create small, dense, harmful LDL particles." It has been shown that a primal diet with significant levels of saturated fat often increases LDL numbers on a lipid panel, but it also increases the particle size from small, dense LDL, which is susceptible to oxidation, to a very-low-density LDL, which is large and fluffy and not as susceptible to oxidation. Very-low-density LDL is precisely the particle type we want for optimal health of both the heart and the brain. These people should eat a ketogenic primal diet if they have this allele. These people would also be wise to limit all dairy intake. I am no fan of any dairy in any diet, but if you have this allele even small amounts can cause massive changes to our hormones, our methylation patterns, and to the epigenetic switches on our genes. Cathome went on to say, "The only rare cases of coronary calcification improvement on EBCT [electron-beam computed tomography heart scan] at a coronary heart website were the uncommon participants on a lower carb, HIGH SATURATED FAT intake." ApoE4 appears to make us exquisitely more sensitive to diet, exercise, fats, carbs, and environmental toxicants. This is why the Primal Rx recommends a ketogenic version of the primal template in higher risk patients. The data I gave you here likely will never be uttered by today's conventional wisdom. I think this advice is way ahead of the curve and firmly based in understanding of evolutionary biology of why natural selection chose some of us to have this allele.

23andme.com is a website that provides single nucleotide polymorphism (SNPs) testing of your entire genome for about $1,000. It gives the following statistics for APO E4 allele.

APOE variant frequencies in Europeans

Genotype Frequency

- ε2/ε2 0.4%
- ε2/ε3 13.7%
- ε3/ε3 63.9%
- ε2/ε4 1.3%
- ε3/ε4 19.0%
- ε4/ε4 1.7%

Data from Lahoz et al (2001).

It should be noted that while there is evidence that the APOE ε4 variant may be associated with higher LDL cholesterol levels, consistent associations have not been demonstrated for coronary heart disease or response to statins.This data comes directly from their website emails they send out to subscribers who carry this allele.

9. Lipoprotein particles (LPA) are small particles containing cholesterol and can be damaging to the arteries if levels are high. LPA particle testing shows a 25-50 percent increase in heart disease risk in those who have elevated levels due to the rapid, progressive development of calcific plaque formation in both coronary and aortic arteries. The main reason I do not advocate testing for this particle is that if one eats a Paleolithic template it removes cardiac risk. If you eat well, you don't have to worry about heart disease. Those with elevated LPA particle size should eat a ketogenic Paleolithic diet very low in carbohydrates and dairy to offset their risks. This is precisely what I recommend in the Primal Rx for heart disease, as well.

10. A word about advanced vertical auto profile (VAP) hacking here is good, too. If you do not opt for a nuclear magnetic resonance (NMR) particle analysis and go with a cheaper VAP, you must be aware that they may identify large fluffy LDLs, but it may not actually be accurate. This occurs because of measuring assumptions done in the VAP. It appears to be a flaw in the VAP methodology. A better way of analyzing this whether you really have very-low-density LDL is to summate subtractions of LDL 3 and LDL 4, then divide that number by your real LDL (not the calculated LDL). That gives you portions of small, dense LDL and is much more accurate than just relying on the VAP's Particle A size. This is why many people choose a NMR over a VAP. If you know about this, you can garner more information from your VAP to guide you, or you can opt for an NMR analysis.

THE PRIMAL RX FOR CARDIAC HEALTH IS TO EAT A PALEOLITHIC TEMPLATE THAT MATCHES YOUR RISKS!

REFERENCES

1. http://www.medicalnewstoday.com/articles/233486.php
2. http://www.mayoclinic.com/health/mens-health/MC00013/NSECTIONGROUP=2
3. http://www.mayoclinic.com/health/womens-health/WO00014/NSECTIONGROUP=2
4. Kenjirou Okamoto, Tetsuya Kakuma, Satoshi Fukuchi, Takayuki Masaki, Toshiie Sakata, Hironobu Yoshimatsu "Sterol regulatory element binding protein (SREBP)-1 expression in brain is affected by age but not by hormones or metabolic changes." Brain Research 1081 (2006) 19–27
5. Steen, et al, Misinformation in the medical literature: What role do error and fraud play? J. Med. Ethics 2011;37:498-503.
6. 13. Vaccarino V, Bremner JD, Kelley ME. JUPITER: a few words of caution. Circ Cardiovasc Qual Outcomes. 2009;2(3):286-288.
7. Ridker PM, Danielson E, Fonseca FA; et al, JUPITER Study Group. Rosuvastatin to prevent vascular events in men and women with elevated C-reactive protein. N Engl J Med. 2008;359(21):2195-2207
8. Michel de Lorgeril MD et al, Cholesterol Lowering, Cardiovascular Diseases, and the Rosuvastatin-JUPITER Controversy A Critical Reappraisal Arch Intern Med. 2010;170(12):1032-1036.
9. http://healthydietsandscience.blogspot.com/2012/01/jupiter-statin-trial-biased-sham.html?spref=tw
10. http://www.sciencedaily.com/releases/2012/01/120120184528.htm

Chapter Ten

AUTOIMMUNITY AND THE LEAKY GUT

CONVENTIONAL WISDOM ABOUT AUTOIMMUNITY

Autoimmune diseases are the black box of medicine, remaining in its blind spot because medicine refuses to look at autoimmune disease from a new perspective. Allopathic medicine does not realize how significantly the gut affects the brain or the immune systems, but once they do it will revolutionize medical advancements.

The gut is the battlefront for most Neolithic diseases, as it is the most significant way we interact with our environment . First, you must realize that many doctors have never even heard the term "leaky gut syndrome." There is no diagnosis of leaky gut in any medical textbook because the connections between the gut and the brain are not well studied by medicine. Physicians, however, do learn about "altered guts" in ICU conditions. So if you remind them of this fact you might make some headway with them. If your doctor worked in an ICU during their training they will be quite familiar with gut health in relation to severe malnutrition, burns, bacterial LPS endotoxemia, and in long term total parenteral nutrition (nutrient IVs), all of which lead to a breakdown in the intestinal brush border. The interesting thing is that few doctors seem to realize this disease shows itself far more commonly in our clinics than it does in the ICU. I believe it is the most common syndrome I see in my neurosurgery clinic today. I also believe medicine will soon link gut health with disease because the current gastroenterology literature is now reaching into this area of science. Gut health affects every system in the body.

Inflammatory bowel disease (IBD) and Crohn's disease deserve special mention because conventional wisdom says neither is tied to diet, despite the large amount of currently published evidence. If you have one of these diseases, you would be wise to immediately employ an autoimmune Paleo diet that eliminates all grain, dairy, and legumes.

RISKS ASSOCIATED WITH LEAKY GUT TO BE AWARE OF:

A. Foods high in the glycemic index, and most dairy products, raw or pasteurized

B. Foods high in refined flours, processed foods with low fiber content

C. Chronic caffeine use

D. Excessive use of alcohol or long-term use or abuse of antibiotics for any reason

E. Chronic use of drugs such as aspirin or ibuprofen (all NSAIDs), and all proton pump inhibitors

F. Mercury-laden foods or any environmental toxins

G. Any disease that causes an altered consciousness (trauma, delirium, dementia, stroke)

H. Chronic or acute food allergies, severe food poisoning, vitamin D levels below 20

I. Burns, excessive training, malnutrition, asthma, eczema, aphthous ulcers (canker sores), pemphigus (skin blistering), lupus, diabetes, and obesity

DISEASES LINKED TO LEAKY GUT

1. Inflammatory bowel diseases such as Crohn's, ulcerative colitis, multiple sclerosis, rheumatoid arthritis, and Hashimoto's thyroiditis

2. Diverticulitis (also very high 6:3 ratios), GERD, and eosinophilic esophagitis

3. Fibromyalgia is an inflammatory disorder that can be screened for with a visual contrast sensitivity test. Our fat cells store these neurotoxins, and when they are released they circulate through fat-containing tissues, wreaking havoc. Producers of these toxins include:

- dinoflagellates, such as Pfiesteria, ciguatera and chattonella;
- fungi, including stachybotrys and fusarium;
- bacteria, such as pseudomonas fluorescens;

- spirochetes, including Lyme disease-causing borrelia;
- blue-green algae, such as rapidly reproducing microcystis and cylindrospermopsis.

4. Degenerative disc disease of the spine and inflammatory spondyloarthropthy; cluster headaches

5. Multiple sclerosis, ALS, Alzheimer's disease, Parkinson's disease, migraines, and atypical headaches

6. Overtraining and adrenal fatigue leading to low 24-hour cortisol; changes in normal diurnal rhythm

7. Eating disorders, especially binge eating disorders triggered by modified gliadin protein in wheat

8. Depression, schizophrenia, bipolar disorder, autism spectrum disorders

9. Heart disease is primarily caused by a leaky gut leading to low HDL and elevated small, dense LDL.

10. Dental caries and periodontal disease are tied to oxidized plasma

11. Obesity is an inflammatory condition of the brain from a leaky gut and elevated IL-6 and leptin levels.

12. Osteoporosis and HIV infection. It appears HIV gains easy access to the brain from the GI tract. Many physicians know it is a neurotrophic virus, but many do not know that it gains access through our GI tract, where it replicates in the mucosa and overwhelms the liver's defenses. This allows it entry into the circulation, which carries it into the brain to cause the major changes allopathic medicine commonly recognizes. HIV seems to really lower IGF-1 and growth hormone secretion to cause sarcopenia.

13. Gallbladder disease is a disease related to high-carb, low-fat dieting that causes a vitamin K2 deficiency.

14. Chronic constipation from dysbiosis in the gut, specifically in the colon.

HOW DO WE TREAT IT? THE LEAKY GUT EPI-PALEO RX FOR AUTOIMMUNITY

1. It's simple, eat a dairy-free version of the Paleolithic diet and add polyphenol-rich vegetables and lots of leafy green vegetables. It would be advisable to make them all organic to avoid pesticides that could cause a secondary Neolithic disease, such as diabetes, from atrazine toxicity.

2. The Spectracell Comprehensive Nutritional Panel is an excellent baseline test, as is the Essential & Metabolic Fatty Acids Analysis (EMFA) by Genova Diagnostics .

3. The hydrogen breath test is a simple test commonly used to screen for small intestinal bacterial overgrowth (SIBO).

A. A hydrogen breath test can be used to diagnose several conditions: H. pylori infection, carbohydrate malabsorption (fructose or lactose), and SIBO.

B. SIBO Breath Test: Breath testing measures the hydrogen and methane gas produced by bacteria in the small intestine, which is diffused into the blood, and then into the lungs for expiration. Hydrogen and methane are gases produced by bacteria, not by humans. The gas is graphed over the small intestine transit time of two or three hours and compared to a baseline. Patients drink a sugar solution of glucose or lactulose after a two-day preparatory diet. The diet removes much of the food that would feed the bacteria, allowing for a clear reaction to the sugar drink.

Two types of tests may be used, lactulose or glucose. I strongly recommend you go to siboinfo.com to learn more about SIBO and the newer research that is being done in this growing area!

The intestinal brush border of our digestive tract is akin to the "motor of our Ferrari," responsible for the multiple organ failures we see in critical illnesses. If you read the gastroenterology literature from the last 10 years, you'll realize the battle for many organs is fought in the gut. The gut mucosa that lines the small intestines produces various acute phase proteins, gut hormones, and cytokines that affect mucosal health as well as the function and integrity of remote organs and tissues. The role of the intestinal mucosa in inflammatory and metabolic responses to sepsis and endotoxemia has become very apparent to researchers during the past decade. The intestinal brush border also appears to be a common origin for most autoimmune diseases.

HASHIMOTO'S HYPOTHYROIDISM

The most commonly known autoimmune disease from a leaky gut is Hashimoto's thyroiditis. Hashimoto's today makes up 95 percent of clinical cases of hypothyroidism. In the Epi-paleo Rx, Hashimoto's is a gateway diagnosis for future development of many different autoimmune diseases, all of which are preceded by a leaky gut. When a patient comes to me with elevated thyroid-stimulating hormone (TSH), a diagnostic marker for hypothyroidism, and the thyroid peroxidase (TPO) or thyroglobulin (TGB) antibodies, which signal an autoimmune thyroid condition, I get very concerned. When the patient is a woman of childbearing age, I am even more concerned. Autoimmune disorders occur more frequently in women than men because women are more sensitive to inflammation. This is because leptin is higher in women of childbearing age and it is an inflammatory IL-6 analogue. In Hashimoto's, the initial attack to the thyroid gland can be by anti-transglutaminase autoantibodies developed in celiac disease or other leaky gut etiologies. Celiac disease may be the initial autoimmune trigger for many other autoimmune diseases and allergies. I believe any leaky gut etiology can cause the problem, hence we need to protect our gut lining from all pathological inflammation.

AUTISM

Autism has been associated with autoimmunity in the mother and placental abnormalities. You might be surprised to learn high concentrations of transglutaminase are found in the placenta, which acts as the gut lining for the fetus. It also appears from recent data that supplemental folic acid in grain products may contribute to the development of leaky gut, altered methylation patterns, and increased inflammation in the fetus' developing brain. As a result, vitamin D and progesterone levels drop in the fetal brain, setting the stage for poor wiring and connection. Other research shows eggs from an older mother, and a mother's low vitamin D and placental progesterone status are critical pieces to understanding the complexities of how autistic spectrum disorders develop. This may help explain why this disorder is becoming more common today: Women are having children later in life, eat a grain-based diet supplemented with folic acid, have low vitamin D levels, and have low progesterone due to inflammation from a chronic leaky gut hindering conversion of pregnenolone to progesterone.

LAB DATA TO REVIEW

Refer back the chapter on lab tests and reread the VAP section to assess a leaky gut. Clues for leaky gut are low HDL, low vitamin D, altered sex steroid hormones, elevated HS-CRP, elevated ferritin, elevated cytokine levels, elevated homocysteine, or a missing gallbladder. Potassium and your blood pressure could also be quite low. This is a sign the aldosterone axis, which regulates sodium balance, fluid volume, and blood pressure, is off, which is often associated with a leaky gut. Some people will also have severe abdominal bloating. I have seen women with guts that can expand in a few weeks to look like they are six months pregnant. This is a sign that your diet is loaded with something your gut lining cannot tolerate. This is when I strongly suggest cutting all dairy, nightshades, and birth control pills. I have found these three are the biggest offenders. Low B12 is also a sign your gut is the problem. If your B12 is below 1000 pg/mL, you need to reassess what you are doing.

Muscle-skeletal pain is often linked to a leaky gut because of several clinical possibilities, including altered magnesium, potassium, and sodium levels, leptin resistance, low hormone levels that decrease lean muscle mass, or low vitamin D.

The cytokines IL1-beta, IL-8, and IL-12 are often tied to a leaky gut diagnosis. A special point needs to be made about IL-12. It is a cytokine associated with leptin resistance and autoimmunity and, in my opinion, is the reason why autoimmunity is more common in women than in men. This is because leptin is higher in women than men due to childbearing. Administration of IL-12 to people suffering from autoimmune disease has been shown to worsen the autoimmune condition because it induces a pro-inflammatory response. In contrast, treatment of mice with IL-12-specific antibodies ameliorated the disease.

The inflammation due to IL-8 is tied directly to the altered cortisol levels and the disruption of the circadian cycle of cortisol. IL-8 is so important that its presence with hepatitis C signifies interferon resistance. This fact is lost on many hepatologists, but the implications are huge when treating leaky gut. IL-8 increases all kinds of cytokines, eventually leading to severe elevations of IL-1beta. IL-1beta is linked to the development of systemic inflammation and multiple sclerosis, rheumatoid arthritis, and Hashimoto's. I have seen the worst cases in women with hepatitis C because they have a leaky gut that cannot be cured due to the ongoing inflammation stimulated by the viral infection. There are some new treatments coming, such as protease inhibitors and pyrimadine inhibitors, but we do not know the long-term effects of these treatments as yet. The protease inhibitors recently approved attack a hepatitis C virus enzyme the virus needs to make new copies of itself. Each of the drugs brings virus replication to a near halt. The unfortunate thing is they have to be used in combination because hepatitis C quickly becomes resistant to them. They also have a very steep side-effect profile. One has to accept this because the hepatitis C virus raises the risk of many Neolithic diseases.

LEAKY GUT RX FOR AUTOIMMUNITY PREVENTION

A. Use grass-fed bones to make a bone broth with coconut oil. Make sure the bones have meat, cartilage, or tendons on them. I like cuts through the joints because it has more L-glutamine than just long bones. This is a core treatment for any leaky gut. Glutamine decreases IL-4 in the brush border to restore health. This is the most critical step in leaky gut repair. If your IL-4 levels are elevated, you know you have a leaky gut for sure. For example, I have yet to test a diabetic who did not have elevated IL-4 levels. The effect of the broth is so brisk that when the body is facing a lipo-polysacharide (LPS) bacterial infection, the medium-chain trigclycerides (MCT) in the coconut oil will re establish brush border integrity. This is but another reason why coconut oil and MCT oils are critical elements to the Epi-paleo Rx

B. Use non-GMO coconut oil as the main fat in the diet until the syndrome is reversed. MCTs significantly blunt pro-inflammatory cytokines, such as TNF-alpha, IL-18, macrophage inflammatory protein-2, and monocyte chemoattractant protein-1 in the ileum. In addition, research showed the mRNA expression of the IgA-stimulating cytokine IL-10 in the ileum and Peyer's patches was significantly greater in those using MCT.

C. Use probiotics liberally if the patient is conscious and not in ICU. Use fermented foods first before going to live culture additives. Examples are sauerkraut, pickles, kimchi, kombucha, yogurt, kefir, artichoke, and horseradish.

D. Consider use of probiotic additives with Lactobacillus acidophilus, Bifido Bacteria, and Saccharomyces Boulardi,

E. You might also supplement with fructo-oligosaccharides (FOS) powders and supplements. These compounds are found naturally in the foods mentioned above in part C, but one also can buy FOS. FOS helps feed the probiotic bacteria in part D, allowing them to flourish and replace the bacteria that foster inflammation at the brush border.

F. Consider supplementing with L-glutamine. Sir Hans Krebs, famous for discovering the Krebs cycle, also found that glutamine improves functioning of the intestinal brush border and the gut-associated lymphoid tissue (GALT), the immune system of the digestive tract. Glutamine is critical for immune regulation of intestinal IgA, antibodies that attack viral and bacterial pathogens in saliva, tears, and in mucous. Glutamine also normalizes cytokines associated with allergies. (Kudsk et al. 2000). (Fukatsu et al. 2001) Also, MCTs slow down the immune response in the brush border, reducing inflammation and encouraging upregulation of IgA production, a protection from bacterial or fungal invasion. Vitamin A further prevents the decline in IgA and is a cofactor in the conversion of LDL cholesterol to pregnenolone. This is another reason why pregnenolone, progesterone, and DHEA levels are low in autoimmune disease and leaky gut, and why these people tend to suffer with low cortisol and adrenal fatigue. My belief is that adrenal fatigue is a condition of sub-acute leaky gut syndrome. I believe serious autoimmune disease is the end result of chronic intestinal inflammation, and we can use hormonal responses to tell us where we're heading. If these inflammatory responses are allowed to chronically feed forward, it leads to massive local and systemic damage. Since it is clear these inflammatory responses are reactions to chronic gut irritants, it suggests the process can be stopped and reversed. I believe this is precisely what Wahls discovered when she reversed her own multiple sclerosis.

G. Other supplements you might use to combat this syndrome: Aloe vera at 2 teaspoons (10 ml) three times a day. This is a major natural fiber, however, and is NOT to be used with Crohn's, ulcerative colitis, or intestinal blockages. You might also use 600 mg of N-acetyl-cysteine (NAC) in combination with 1,000-2,000 mg of vitamin C. You might even consider vitamin C infusions intravenously. NAC is the precursor for glutathione, one of our body's main antioxidants. Some people with severe disease may need intravenous glutathione treatment. Low glutathione levels also correlate with positive serum antibodies for diseases that are not active. A glutathione deficiency compromises our ability to keep old viruses dormant and fight off bacteria. This is why so many people test positive for Epstein-Barr virus (EBV), cytomegalovirus (CMV), HHV-6 herpes virus, mycoplasma, and Chlamydia Pneumoniae when they have leaky gut or autoimmune disease.

H. Clinical Pearls: My clinical beliefs are that glutathione can stop the replication of any intracellular microbe, including HHV6, Chlamydia Pneumoniae, and mycoplasma. I learned this from several anti-aging physicians who found that some of their patients were becoming virus free after using undenatured whey protein for approximately six months. This type of whey protein helps restore glutathione levels. It also is effective for weight loss because it improves leptin status. This information is vital to HIV patients, who all have leaky guts, and is a very cheap and easy way for them to increase their levels of glutathione and assist their antiretroviral drugs to keep viral titers low. It actually works well for many viral diseases, such as Hepatitis C. The nice thing about this protocol is that you can do it at home for the most part, and you can assess whether it is working or not.

Increasing your glutathione levels works even better when you're optimizing your uric acid defense system, too. Uric acid is a natural antioxidant, accounting for up to 60 percent of the free radical scavenging activity in human blood (Ames et al., 1981). Uric acid scavenges superoxide hydroxyl radical and single oxygen atoms. (Ames et al., 1981; Davies et al., 1986). Uric acid appears to help remove superoxide by preventing the degradation of superoxide dismutase (SOD). SOD is the enzyme responsible for chemically cleansing superoxide from the cell (Pacher et al., 2007). Removing superoxide helps prevent the formation of peroxynitrite, a mitochondrial toxin. This is important for neurodegenerative diseases and multiple sclerosis. The driver of this whole process, however, is the leaky gut.

People with leaky guts tend to have low levels of intracellular uric acid and glutathione. You should also know that aging is associated with low glutathione and uric acid.

Glutathione is a critical test to run on people with leaky gut or autoimmunity. So are B12 and folate levels. It's really important to know what your levels of folate and B12 are prior to taking any glutathione precursors, as a B12 or folate deficiency will cause glutathione deficiency. This is why I advocate high B12 levels through diet, sublingually, or intramuscular injection if your gut is too damaged for you to absorb it orally. Most people with gut problems can't, and this is why their leaky gut persists. Do B12 drops first and then folate. You can monitor this at home by observing your urine color after taking a glutathione precursor from any source. If your urine turns a rose or reddish color, then you are excreting too much B12 and the glutathione is going to waste. If your urine is greenish, you are depleted in folate and need to increase that before you add any more glutathione.

The more severe the autoimmune disease the worse the glutathione deficits. This is why we see a strong relationship between low glutathione levels and autism spectrum disorders, depression, and neurodegenerative disorders. Toxins accumulate when glutathione levels are low. So just getting rid of the toxin offers little protection if you are not reestablishing glutathione levels with diet and supplementation. When faced with this problem, another clinical pearl is an ALCAT food allergy test. They are typically worthless in my opinion, but the one time they are useful is when you test positive for more than 50 to 75 percent of foods. Most providers do not know what to make of this, but it is a sign that you have very low glutathione levels. So this is a tip you need to fix this pathway before jumping into the dietary modification. If done correctly, you can see major improvement in seven days. Supplements that work well in these cases are: NAC, alpha-lipoic acid, milk thistle or fever few, curcumin, and acetyl L-carnitine. In addition, glutathione is essential in supporting and maintaining the immune system. This is especially critical because the highest level of glutathione and disease-fighting immune cells are found in the gut. Evolution designed it that way because that is where the battle of survival begins. It's where food first interacts with the immune system. Per serving, asparagus, avocados, squash, okra, cauliflower, broccoli, artichokes, burdock root, jicama, spinach, walnuts, garlic, and raw ripe red tomatoes have the highest glutathione content compared to other vegetables, and are particularly rich dietary sources of glutathione. They should be what you put in your broths.

LEAKY GUT LINKS TO IMMUNITY AND PAIN CONTROL SYSTEMS

When glutathione levels are low patients complain of poor well-being; they feel bad. This is a sign the leaky gut has likely gotten to the brain via the vagus nerve. This raises leptin levels and lowers alpha-melanocyte-stimulating hormone (MSH), a hormone secreted by the pituitary gland that regulates pigmentation, eating behavior, and energy homeostasis. High leptin gradually progress to leptin resistance and inflammation. This is how inflammation is passed from the intestinal brush border to the brain. Often these people report weight loss resistance. When MSH decreases its effect on the immune system is interesting, which I learned about long ago from the neurobiology of HIV patients. Remember, HIV is a neurotropic virus that best gains access to our bodies via our GI tract. As MSH falls and leptin rises, the endorphin pathways of the brain decline fast. This is what causes that feeling of being sick. Simultaneously, levels of ACTH from the brain fall. ACTH stimulates the release of adrenal hormones, and these people become chronically fatigued with high levels of unexplained pain. The endorphin pathways comprise a class of at least 25 neural hormones that have vast actions in many systems of our body. They are made in the both the central and peripheral nervous systems, and in other places, such as the adrenal glands. Diseases linked to a leaky gut also are always associated with low levels of endorphins and endocabinoids, substances that play a role in appetite, memory, and pain. The HIV researchers in the late 1980s found that 95 percent of our immune cells have receptors for both endorphins and endocabinoids. In essence, sufficient levels of these feel-good chemicals help us mount an appropriate immune response to a toxin or pathogen, and low levels make us feel sick. This is even more pronounced when the inflammation is chronic, as in autoimmunity, cancer, mental illness, or viral diseases.

The ways we can increase these two systems are to stop the chronic inflammation and stop the leakiness at the brush border. Often, that process takes time, even after the diet is solved. Another tool is high-intensity interval training (HIIT), an exercise strategy that alternates bursts of short intense anaerobic exercise with less-intense recovery periods for 10 to 20 minutes. Meditation or acupuncture are other ways to improve this downside of inflammation. A few others ideas that may surprise you are making your environment cold and eating pure chocolate without mycotoxins. Resveratrol and the polyphenols in chocolate are nothing short of amazing.

Another way not well known or used by conventional medicine is low-dose naltrexone therapy (LDN). This blocks the endorphin receptors, stimulating the body to produce its own endogenous endorphins. The effect of LDN only lasts a short period of time. In people with mild cases of leaky gut it is usually more effective. Those with more serious chronic inflammation tend to have no response to this treatment. These are all options to consider when you have lost your sense of well-being or have chronic lowered immunity. People who respond best often have low levels of vitamin D and moderate IL-6 levels as well.

People with serious skin manifestations of leaky gut, such as psoriasis or eosinophilic folliculitis (an itchy rash typically associated with HIV), should consider NAC because it directly blocks IL-4, a main factor in the production of IgE antibodies. IgE antibodies are made in hay fever, asthma, anaphylactic shock, and atopic skin diseases. If the asthma is severe, one can measure the amount of nitric oxide directly in the expired air and it will be elevated. When this happens you also see drops in vitamin D. This is why these diseases seem to peak in fall and winter-most people do not have good stores of vitamin D. Vitamin D levels are chronically low partly because of the beliefs imprinted on us by dermatologists to shield our skin from sunlight with sunscreens. Moreover, lack of antioxidants is found in emphysema, chronic obstructive pulmonary disease, and cystic fibrosis. (Corradi et al. 2001) NAC will form glutathione and combine with nitric oxide to create nitrosothiols, compounds related to the dilation of blood vessels and oxygenation of the body. This binding reduces the inflammatory effects of nitric oxide in the body to limit disease quickly. This is also critical for leaky gut. Medicine has yet to make these links. You need to now to protect yourself. They are common mechanisms used in many disease states. Don't worry if you don't understand the science. The bottom line is fix your gut and disease goes away.

I. Magnesium. Magnesium, zinc, and CoQ10 are all major cofactors in the stress response and used up quickly in leaky gut syndrome. To compensate, supplement with 400-1,200 mg of magnesium at night, 25-75 mg of zinc a day, and 400-1,200 mg of Co Q10 a day (depending upon severity of the disease). They can all be replaced with supplementation, but seek first to get them in your food. If you have an intolerance to magnesium, consider an epsom salt bath three times a week to replenish magnesium levels and add sulfur to your cartilage. This is a key treatment option for those with degenerative disc disease who have low vitamin D and low sex steroid levels. I use this one a lot in my spine clinic.

J. Consider liberal use of omega-3 supplements or krill oil, or increase your astaxathin to 4-8 mg a day), and increase your intake of omega-3 laden foods, such as fresh fish.

K. Consider deglycyrrhizinated licorice root (DGL). The dose here is 500 mg extract (10:1) three times a day. This is an adaptogen that normalizes cortisol levels, but this form is also extremely helpful for leaky gut because it does not have any of the side effects of using whole licorice, such as causing low potassium, low sodium, edema, high blood pressure, and palpitations.

L. For people with resistant leaky gut, ask your mom if you were breast-fed and for how long. If the answer is not at all or very little, then consider the use of colostrum as a consistent supplement. Bodybuilders have long used it to allow them to overtrain while closing the permeability of their brush border. It is that effective. Many people do not realize that exercise can open your gut to inflammation. The reason colostrum works so well is because it loaded with proline. The proline-rich peptides in colostrum have been shown to support the thymus gland, and may help calm an overactive immune system and stimulate an underactive immune system.

Also, you can be tested for the following celiac antibodies:

- Immunoglobulin A
- Deamidated gliadin
- Tissue transglutamine IgA

One must remember that the testing commonly done for gluten/gliadin intolerance is not as accurate because of the modifications made to wheat, which is outlined in the literature. So a negative test does not mean you are free and clear. This is why elimination diets tell you much more clinically, in my opinion. There is no good biologic reason to eat any grain.

M. The Dr. Shoemaker protocol for fibromyalgia, Lyme disease, and chronic fatigue patients (chronicneurotoxins.com): Perform the visual contrast sensitivity (VCS) test first. This test assesses optic nerve function in relation to contrast, which assesses the effects of neurotoxins on the patient's system. It evaluates two sets of nerves in the eye that differentiate between white, black, and gray on a gray background. It has been found that a person with biotoxin-associated illness will not be able to identify the various patterns. Failure to successfully complete this test is a strong indicator of a biotoxin illness. Though it is possible for a person impacted by biotoxins to pass the test (a false negative result), this occurs only in about 8 percent of test subjects. Thus, the VCS test supports diagnosis in about 92 percent of affected people. False positives are quite rare.

There are specific genotypes associated with susceptibility to biotoxins. Approximately 25 percent of the population has a genetic inability to naturally clear biotoxins. Patients who have this genetic predisposition will need extra help from their physicians to clear the toxin using two drugs. The genetic test is called HLA DR, and it is more commonly known as a test that provides insight into organ rejection after a transplant operation. One can use an interpretation guide written by the protocol's founder, Ritchie Shoemaker, MD, which correlates the HLA DR findings to specific conditions that may be associated with multiple biotoxin diseases. The biotoxins can bind to Toll receptors in the gut, in fat cells, or in cells that line blood vessels, resulting in immune responses and inflammatory processes. Matrix metallo-peptidase 9 (MMP9) is a superb marker for the presence of excess cytokines production from any inflammatory disease, and is rarely used. I use this one for spine hacks.

MMP9 may be responsible for delivering inflammatory compounds to the brain, which causes plaque formations similar to those seen in multiple sclerosis. In Lyme disease, MMP9 levels may skyrocket as the result of treatment with antibiotics and bacterial die-off, in what is commonly referred to as a Herxheimer reaction. We also see this with candida die-off, for which MMP9 can also be followed. During this reaction, the symptoms usually get more severe. Cholestyramine, a drug used to lower cholesterol, can often mitigate the effect by binding the biotoxins circulating in the fat. If you are dealing with a Lyme disease diagnosis based on the HLA DR array, you must first kill the spirochete bacteria and then go after the neurotoxin that causes the pain and obesity associated with Lyme. If you give a Lyme-infected person antibiotics and they are not HLA-susceptible, recovery is generally uneventful because they can clear the toxin by themselves without the help of cholestyramine or Actos, a drug that helps control blood sugar. Actos liberates neurotoxins from the fat so cholestyramine can bind and eliminate it.

An increase in cytokines may also trigger autoimmunity if the process is chronic. There are three types of antibodies observed in those with biotoxin-associated illnesses. These antibodies are to myelin (the protective sheath around nerve cells), gliadin (a protein found in gluten), and cardiolipin (which impacts circulation in the small blood vessels).

There also may be notable increases in C3a and C4a. The "C" stands for "complement," and C3 and C4a are proteins that work with antibodies and activate immunity. There is a significant difference in C3a and C4a levels between controls and in people with Lyme or mold toxicity. In fact, C4a levels become elevated, often as early as 12 hours after a tick bite. In the case of those with a mold-susceptible HLA type, C4a significantly increases within four hours after re-exposure to a moldy environment. C4a can be a

helpful marker in determining whether or not a remediated home is still a danger for someone with mold biotoxin susceptibility.

WHERE DOES LEPTIN ENTER THE PICTURE FOR THESE DISEASES?

The reason I became interested in these diseases was two-fold. One, as a pine surgeon, a lot of people are referred to me with axial mechanical spinal ain (low back pain). Often, many have these other diseases and not spine disease. Two, all these diseases are tied to leptin biochemistry and I learned to cure myself of a leptin illness, so I now happen to know a lot about how this issue connects to so many Neolithic diseases. This will become much clearer to you when you read the last chapter of this book.

When neural biotoxins elevate cytokines and inflammation, leptin levels rise. When leptin increases, alpha MSH in the hypothalamus decreases. Shoemaker found any biotoxin exposure decreases alpha MSH, which is associated with increased pain and a propensity to gain weight. So with these diseases we see leptin increase, alpha MSH decrease, and patients become obese and very resistant to weight loss. When I learned about these links, it immediately made me realize how important leptin was in many diseases. These patients also become very sensitive to any painful stimuli.

Alpha MSH is the key finding in these neural biotoxin diseases as it controls the biotoxin pathways. With Lyme disease, chronic fatigue, mold illness, and any other biotoxin illness, regardless of the source of the biotoxin, we see a reduction in alpha MSH in 95-98 percent of patients. This has huge implications for other Neolithic disease processes we will look at in the last chapter.

When alpha MSH levels are low, people also develop sleep disorders, chronic pain, and leaky gut, which increase inflammation even more. Because of this, their recovery from illness is often delayed. These patients may develop multiple antibiotic resistant coagulase-negative staph colonization (MARCoNS), although most doctors don't recognize this. When I see this on a pre-surgical screen I realize we might have a large pain management issue brewing before the surgery even occurs. These patients tend to have frequent thirst as a result of low anti-diuretic hormone (ADH), which can be associated with large blood losses from surgery. They also have low libido due to low sex hormone levels caused by inflammation at the hypothalamus. All these can be found with simple hormone testing. Alpha

MSH is involved in the production of melatonin and endorphins. This is why sleep and pain are involved in these disorders.

This resulting lack of natural endorphins increases pain perception. When a physician says there is not disease called fibromyalgia, I get very angry. There is a clear pathophysiology present, but modern medicine has not tied the known information of these diseases together with the hypothalamic wiring in the brain. I came to understand these diseases by first understanding leptin and its relationship to inflammation.

There is also another facet to the alpha MSH story. The higher it is, the less pain we have. It appears that light and geothermal cycles regulate our MSH levels, and this is also tied to the leptin receptor because of evolution. The real reason is quite surprising. I believe it is to protect us from recurrent ice ages, which we have faced in our pasts. I will discuss this relationship and its implications for us in an upcoming chapter.

Understanding the nuances of the evolutionary biology behind Lyme disease, fibromyalgia, and mold toxicity explains the many muscle aches and pains these patients suffer. It also underscores why they can't exercise well and or lose weight, even if they push through their pain. The lack of understanding of the pathophysiology behind these diseases is why patients have become uber-frustrated with conventional medicine. I hope now you understand it enough so you can navigate around what your doctors tell you without feeling bad about it. They just do not see what you now know. I do not want this disconnect in your relationship with your doctor to drive your cortisol levels higher, further lower your alpha MSH, and increase your pain!

Alpha MSH also regulates the protective cytokine responses in the blood, skin, digestive tract, and respiratory membranes. Low alpha MSH results in cortisol abnormalities and fluctuations in ACTH, which regulates adrenal function. People with chronic adrenal fatigue often have biotoxin disease and rarely know it. Many who have a sustained leaky gut are susceptible to adrenal fatigue because of increased leptin and decreased alpha MSH. This is why people with adrenal fatigue are always tired, can't lose weight, and sleep poorly. It has very little to do with carbohydrate intake or a glucose deficiency.

One way to assess this is to test your alpha MSH levels at the same time as your C4a levels. If Lyme is suspected, your infectious disease physician can run a CD57 test to see if you are chronically infected. If you are, you need to make sure the spirochete is killed before you proceed. An informed

infectious disease physician or a primary care physician with Lyme train[illegible] is critical in helping you navigate back to optimal health.

TREATMENT:

1. If you are dealing with acute Lyme, it must be treated with th[illegible] weeks of antibiotics. Then you must try to clear the biotoxin from the b[illegible]teria. I strongly suggest you seek an infectious disease physician experien[illegible] treating Lyme disease, fibromyalgia, or chronic fatigue. Ten to 15 mill[illegible] Americans suffer from these often misdiagnosed diseases. Most get labe[illegible] with other diagnoses, such as depression, chronic pain, IBD, etc. W[illegible] Most doctors never learn about the easy visual contrast sensitivity test

This test is akin to a neurosurgeon looking at your optic discs to check for increased intracranial pressure. It is easy, cheap, and takes all of three minutes to administer. In fact, you can give it to yourself. If the result is positive, then you can then begin to get the correct testing to assist your non-believing MD. Once you show him or her the other classic findings, those tests will force action. I see a lot of people who come to me for back pain who have these diseases. I start by asking two questions. 1. Me: "Are you sensitive to bright light?" Patient: "Yes. Especially at night, doctor. Headlights really get me!" 2. Me: "Do your muscles constantly ache?" Patient: "Hell yes, Doc, and especially the day after I do normal physical activities."

After those two I make sure they are not on a statin that can cause the same symptoms, and then I tell them they need to do the VCS. Simple. If they have a positive VCS, I send them to the infectious disease docs, who treat them to remove the toxin or kill the bacteria.

2. Cholestyramine (CSM) is a resin that has been used historically for lowering cholesterol. It is very effective in clearing biotoxins as well. It works within 48 hours of treatment, binding the toxins from the fat. It is very cheap as well. It has a positive charge that binds to a wide range of low molecular weight, negatively charged toxins, and helps shuttle them out of the body through the digestive tract. It is not systemically absorbed. CSM is like a vacuum cleaner that sucks up all the toxins released from your fat cells as treatment protocols proceed. CSM use usually leads to a dramatic fall in C4a levels. If C4a levels rise again while you're on CSM or antibiotics, you must assume the Lyme spirochete, mold, or neurotoxin is not eradicated and still present in your tissues.

3. Treatment for biotoxins may include Actos, a notorious type 2 diabetes drug. Actos was recently black boxed because of its association with an increase in bladder cancer when used over a year. However, one can use it short-term in these diseases to help liberate neurotoxins from the fat cells or the lymphatic system to be cleared by the CSM vacuum cleaner. It has a significant number of physiologic benefits for patients with biotoxin associated illnesses. Actos lowers leptin levels, lowers matrix metallo peptidase 9 (MMP9), lowers vascular endothelial growth factor (VEGF), and positively increases PPAR-gamma, which causes fat cells to empty, all while improving insulin resistance and lowering inflammation. It basically causes our fat cells to dump their toxic contents so CSM can slowly remove them over time. For these diseases, it is precisely how we need to cleanse the fat of toxins. It is one of the most important interventions known in treating biotoxin illnesses, as it seems to block the cytokine storm, or Herxheimer reaction that occurs in 50 percent of Lyme patients. The interesting thing is that Actos will not work if you eat a SAD. It works best if you eats a ketogenic Paleolithic diet because of its effects on leptin and cytokine amplification.

HOW DO I KNOW I AM BETTER?

1. HS-CRP levels approach zero and cytokine panels normalize. Skin clears, asthma resolves, migraines improve, and your muscles stop aching. Your sleep magically improves quickly.

2. You don't have any unusual pain, bloating, indigestion, constipation, or other symptoms consistent with a leaky gut.

3. Intestinal permeability test: This is the simpler of the two lab tests. (The other test is listed next.) You consume a concoction of two non-digestible sugars, lactulose and mannitol, then collect your urine. Testing examines the content of the two sugars. In a healthy gut, mannitol is easily absorbed whereas lactulose is only slightly absorbed. But with intestinal permeability, the lactulose is easily absorbed through the leaking gaps in the intestinal wall. This test can be ordered from Genova Diagnostics (www.genovadiagnostics.com). These tests are rarely used in allopathic medicine, sadly. If you are suffering from a disease linked to leaky gut, it is a great investment in my opinion.

4. Intestinal Barrier Function Test: This is the more comprehensive of the two tests and analyzes a saliva or blood serum sample. It looks

at the immune antibody levels to bacteria, yeast, and the most common food-intolerant dietary proteins (wheat, corn, soy, cow's milk, and egg). The levels of the measured antibodies determine what stage of development you are currently in.

It also looks at the severity of the issues driving your condition, giving you insight into some of the common allergenic foods you should be removing from your diet. This test can be ordered from BioHealth Diagnostics (www.biodia.com)

REFERENCES

1. http://escholarship.umassmed.edu/cgi/viewcontent.cgi?article=1025&context=cts_retreat
2. http://fitfemaleforty.com/2010/11/10/got-leaky-gut/
3. http://pen.sagepub.com/content/29/1/44.abstract
4. http://pen.sagepub.com/content/24/5/270.abstract
5. http://ajpgi.physiology.org/content/286/6/G1081.full
6. http://www.ncbi.nlm.nih.gov/pmc/articles/PMC1420810/
7. Bardella MT, Elli L, Matteis SD, Floriani I, Torri V, Piodi L. Autoimmune disorders in patients affected by celiac sprue and inflammatory bowel disease. Ann Med. 2009;41(2):139-43.
8. Kathy S. Wang, David A. Frank, and Jerome Ritz. Blood, Vol 95 No. 10 pp. 3183:3190 "Interleukin-2 enhances the response of natural killer cells to interleukin-12 through up-regulation of the interleukin-12 receptor and STAT4".
9. Temblay JN, Bertelli E, Arques JL, Regoli M, Nicoletti C. Production of IL-12 by Peyer patch-dendritic cells is critical for the resistance to food allergy, J Allergy Clin Immunol. 2007 Sep;120(3):659-65. Epub 2007 Jun 28.
10. http://www.gutpathogens.com/content/3/1/1

Chapter Eleven

CENTRAL NERVOUS SYSTEM DISEASES OF STROKE, NEURODEGENERATION, AND AGING

From an evolutionary viewpoint, aging is a biologic novelty. Human evolution is based on success at reproduction, not a long life span. Aging has become society's most troubling burden, an issue revealed through the explosive growth of neurodegenerative disorders in the last 120 years. Sadly, my profession does not seem to appreciate the genesis of neurodegenerative disorders, and has no answers to curb their prevalence.

Evolution selects for optimal reproduction; longevity is not its focus. As scientist Peter Gluckman pointed out, "survival later in life will be less strongly selected and thus selection may have compromised health in middle and old age." Consequently, the Epi-paleo Rx needs to be mindful of this perspective, as what was best for us in our younger years might be detrimental as we age. We do not know this to be true as of yet, but our Neolithic minds need to account for this possible pitfall of aging.

We know normal aging increases inflammation, which is correlated with lower conversion of LDL cholesterol to pregnenolone. Low pregnenolone is one of the most common responses we see in aging. This conversion requires vitamin A and the thyroid hormone T3, and we lose the ability to make T3 from T4 first in the gut and then in our cells. As we age we also may notice our LDL levels rise. This, too, is a sign to check for declining pregnenolone. If we find these things together, the best treatment is to add a small dose of T3 to our daily regimen of medications to offset the loss.

One reason we see atherosclerosis increase as we age is because we cannot convert LDL cholesterol to patch the inside of damaged arteries. When conversion rates fall, the cholesterol might stay in our plasma too long and eventually become oxidized, making it a source of atherosclerosis. The small density LDL is profoundly susceptible to this type of reaction. This is why a Paleolithic diet helps mitigate the risks of aging-it is low in foods that generate inflammation and toxicity, thus lowering the risk of arterial disease. The diet is also very high in L-carnosine, which has been shown to increase telomere lengths. If you can keep inflammation low, thus preserving mitochondrial integrity, you have an opportunity to increase your lifespan just by altering your diet.

DOES MTOR AND IGF-1 ACTIVATION ALWAYS SHORTEN LIFE SPAN WITH THE EPI-PALEO RX?

Most longevity research points to decreased lifespan when the two nutrient growth pathways are activated. Those two pathways are mTOR and IGF-1 pathways. The key point is that these studies were performed on older people who had higher levels of inflammation because of their age and their standard diets. Therefore, conclusions made from these studies cannot be generalized to humans who alter their diets. Inflammation is at the seat of aging. Telomere biology shows their lengths are directly tied to the efficiency and integrity of mitochondria, the energy factories in our cells. Much about the Paleolithic diet favors longevity. A longitudinal study (a study of repeated observations over a long period of time) needs to be done because I believe it may show that activating mTOR with high-protein and high-fat diets and increasing IGF-1 levels with protein and carbohydrates may not hurt our longevity, as the research says it might. This is a very real hole in our current science. We do not know this answer and, therefore, I default to what evolutionary biology tells us.

Our knowledge to date says telomere lengths determine cellular fate and the aging process. Shortened telomere lengths in organs correspond to organ degeneration and failure. It's clear the human telomere is our best measuring stick for therapeutic interventions, and the Paleolithic diet has the most advantages for reduce aging and Neolithic disease. The incidences of the diseases we discuss in this chapter rise as humans enter middle age.

With diseases of the brain, heart, and arterial tree, it may be beneficial to favor fats, specifically medium chain triglycerides (MCTs). The common tie between heart disease, atherosclerosis (hardening of the arteries), and neurodegenerative diseases, such as Alzheimer's, is the advanced aging of arteries and poor blood flow to the organs.

Most doctors also advocate the use of statins and warfarin (Coumadin) without any good science to support them. These drugs alter neurons to cause major problems in cognition and allow for calcification of arterial walls.

CONVENTIONAL WISDOM ADVICE FOR STROKES

You need to pay attention to your lipids. Eat a low-fat, high-carbohydrate diet and take your statins and blood pressure medications. I think we will put you on some kind of blood thinner like Coumadin or Pradaxa. You need to exercise more and stop being a lazy slug. People with severe atherosclerosis may have elevated LPA particle sizes, too.

EPI-PALEO RX FOR STROKES

Eat a diet opposite of conventional wisdom advice. This would be a Paleolithic diet laden with MCT oils. You would also be wise to eat carbohydrates low in the glycemic index to keep your particle size large and fluffy. You want to keep your HS-CRP as close to zero as possible, and your Vitamin D levels up. You should not supplement with calcium, and you should eat foods high in vitamin K2, or supplement with it. A Paleolithic diet is the best way for you to limit your risks from all strokes.

There are many kinds of strokes and some have some key features that alter our view of them.

A. Strokes from atherosclerosis and poor blood flow are called ischemic intracranial disease. These need aggressive vitamin K2 replacement and optimization of the sex hormones. If your TSH is high, you would be wise to try to get it between 0.5 to 2.0. You also want to keep your insulin level below 2 and begin an exercise program.

B. Hemorrhagic strokes are caused by weakened and calcified vessels in certain parts of the brain. The best treatment is the addition of high-dose vitamin K2 to your ketogenic Paleolithic diet. Control of your blood pressure is important here, too.

C. Amyloid angiopathy is a brain disorder tied to altered lipid metabolism that leads to fragility of the supporting elements of the brain. These people are susceptible to blood clots in the brain and must eat a strict ketogenic diet high in MCTs, and they must monitor their blood pressure closely. This disorder is often seen with Alzheimer's disease.

D. Subarachnoid hemorrhages are due to ballooning of cerebral vessels at their branch points in the brain. These tend to occur much earlier and life and are deadly. No one really knows the cause but they are associated with changes in the vessel wall, and many believe they are tied to a genetic predisposition. I believe these people can remodel their vessels with high-dose B vitamins, magnesium supplementation, vitamin D3 supplementation, high-dose vitamin K2 supplementation, and maximizing a reduced serum plasma. There is no good proof for this advice because it is not well studied, but all these maneuvers support optimal arterial wall functioning. Limiting PUFAs and trans-fats is critical to avoid weak arterial walls.

ALZHEIMER'S DISEASE

Conventional wisdom advice for Alzheimer's

Many believe Alzheimer's is a genetic disease. Most people are not sure of the cause.

Epi-paleo Rx for Alzheimer's

Alzheimer's disease is a nutritional disease with inflammation at its foundation. You need to eat a complete ketogenic diet loaded in MCT oils and coconut oils. Carbohydrate intake for Alzheimer's has to be the lowest of any diet. These diet changes are critical for success. Of course, the best treatment is prevention by eating well before you get the disease. Diabetics are at a massive risk for developing Alzheimer's disease, which is why rates of Alzheimer's have exploded-the rates of diabetes have exploded, too.

THE ALZHEIMER'S DISEASE CHAIN OF EVIDENCE FOR CAUSATION: GENES OR EPIGENETICS?

The recent announcements about the potential causes of Alzheimer's disease have gained a lot of attention, but what most caught my eye was information about genes tied to lipid metabolism and inflammation. The Alzheimer's jigsaw puzzle is a long way from complete, but emerging information suggest inflammation is the root cause of this condition, and that inflammation is tied to diet. What exactly are those pieces of evidence?

1. Insoluble plaques inside neurons made of a protein called amyloid beta cause Alzheimer's.

These proteins accumulate over time, blocking normal brain signal transmissions and molecule transfers. During this time, the brain becomes susceptible to hemorrhages. As the amyloid proteins accumulate, tau proteins also accumulate, and the two interact chemically to form an insoluble protein called a neurofibrillary tangle, which is classically associated with many neurodegenerative diseases (Alzheimer's, Parkinson's, and mad cow disease are a few).

2. Researchers and clinicians believe your risk of getting Alzheimer's rises dramatically if you carry the Apo E gene. It appears it raises your risk of atherosclerosis, too. In fact, having two copies of the allele raises your risk of developing Alzheimer's 20-fold before the age of 75.

Apo E remove's the build up of amyloid beta and tau proteins before they damage brain cells in a process called apoptosis. Alzheimer's increases apoptosis, slowly destroying the brain.

Protein folding is a process by which the protein assumes its shape. Diseases such as Alzheimer's are believed to be due to protein misfolding. The solubility of proteins determines how they fold. If the protein folds incorrectly, it becomes less soluble. This is why we can visualize tangles under a microscope. Ironically, this points to the presence of Apo E gene being very positive, more proof that genetic determinism is not as important as epigenetics.

3. The third bit of evidence comes from Chris Dobson's lab at Cambridge University in England.

Dobson made 17 small genetic adjustments to the amyloid beta protein in his lab, to make it either more or less soluble. After doing this, he then transferred these genetically altered proteins into the DNA of fruit flies, proving less soluble proteins resulted in shorter-lived flies. So after this experiment, neuroscientists began to ask, why do misfolded proteins show up in elderly brains to begin with?

4. It appears all neurons have internal, quality-control mechanisms that not only detect misfolded proteins, but also prevent misfolding from happening.

Research published in March 2011 from Brown University showed that both parts of this mechanism, the detector and refolder, are functional in diseased brains, but the process is overwhelmed by neurodegenerative changes. Basically, they cannot sustain the maintenance workload of all the amyloid beta proteins being made.

5. The fifth bit of evidence came in April 2011 from Jeffrey Kelly, PhD, at the Scripps Research Institute. Kelly found a chemical forms when cholesterol reacts with ozone. Ozone is a reactive form of oxygen. We refer to it as a free radical. The ozone then attaches to amyloid beta proteins and makes misfolding hundreds of times more likely. Kelly found the ozone came from inflammation generated within the neurons. They linked the etiology of protein misfolding directly to carbohydrate and omega six in the diet, both of which are known to create inflammation. It also tightly links diabetes with Alzheimer's.

6. The last bit of evidence comes from the recent studies on stress and the development of neurodegenerative diseases due to the hormone cortisol. We know that leptin resistance causes diabetes. Chronic leptin resistance progresses to insulin resistance and eventually to adrenal resistance, in which insulin and cortisol are chronically elevated. Chronic cortisol elevation is associated with inflammation. Cortisol is made from pregnenolone. In 2011, work done at the University of California, Irvine pointed to the elevation of cortisol as the main generator of inflammation in diseased neurons. This is what fuels the rise of ozone in the diseased brains of Alzheimer's victims. The elevated cortisol also fuels more protein misfolding, overwhelming the detector and refolding mechanisms in the brain. This accelerates as the disease progresses, and is why we see neurologic decline when the brain is fueled consistently by carbohydrates and PUFAs.

Based upon this evidence we can see this is not a genetic disease but a nutritional disease. The major problem in neurons is the misfolding protein. Because of this, Alzheimer's is now classified as a "proteopathy." A proteopathy is a disease of misfolded proteins. It appears that Alzheimer's disease is caused by several key factors that appear in unison.

The first finding is that people with Alzheimer's have an extreme lack of lipids in the brain, particularly omega-3 fats. It appears the brain needs 25-35 percent of the omega-3 fat DHA to function optimally. We also see upregulation of the IGF-1 pathways and dysregulation of protein signaling, both of which lead to faulty protein folding in the Alzheimer's brain. We used to think Alzheimer's was due to tau proteins causing neurofibrillary tangles, but it is becoming clear the real issue is the remnants of faulty protein folding causing non-functional neurons. The neurons containing these misfolded proteins are toxic and therefore undergo apoptosis. As the process progresses the brain's stem cell supply in the temporal, parietal and frontal lobes becomes exhausted.

It appears this pathologic process uses up the brain's cholesterol stores to make the cortisol fueling the inflammation. So Alzheimer's results in a cholesterol deficiency in the brain! It is no wonder Alzheimer's is growing like mad considering medicine has been trying to drive cholesterol levels into the ground with inflammatory low-fat, high-carb diets. This is why statins are terrible choices for people with neurodegenerative diseases. The inflammation overwhelms the quality-assurance system that ensures proper protein folding, and the end result is the formation of neurofibrillary tangles from insoluble proteins. These insoluble proteins then block the transport of vital ingredients into the brain cells to offset the assault. One of those vital ingredients appears to be cholesterol itself. We now know high insulin levels block LDL cholesterol from entering the brain. It appears repair mechanisms for normal lipid metabolism becomes so imbalanced it induces nerve cells to undergo apoptosis and deplete themselves. This is why, as a neurosurgeon, I see cerebral atrophy on MRI and CT scans in these patients.

In my opinion, based on the information we have today, Alzheimer's is a nutritional disorder.

When it comes to Alzheimer's, researchers hope we can find ways to attack or block the inflammation, the production of ozone reactions, the conversion of cholesterol to cortisol, and encourage the refolding apparatus that evolution provided. Maybe then we can improve protein solubility and even boost the plaque removal mechanism. I have a much simpler and cheaper idea. Why don't we just stop lighting the match for the dynamite?

Maybe we should advocate a ketogenic Paleolithic diet that decreases carbohydrates and lowers omega-6 fatty acids. Since we now know what drives the disease, we know what will slow its progression. Of course, somehow I bet they'd rather make a profitable drug rather than teach people what might really help. After all, no food company makes money unless they are selling the SAD, do they? The choice is yours.

REFERENCES

1. http://www.bmj.com/content/343/bmj.d7671?etoc
2. Kirkwood TB, Austad SN. Why do we age? Nature2000;408:233-8. CrossRefMedline
3. Gluckman PD, Hanson MA, Spencer HG, Bateson P. Environmental influences during development and their later consequences for health and disease: implications for the interpretation of empirical studies. Proc Biol Sci2005;272:671-7.
4. Gluckman PD, Beedle AS, Hanson MA. Principles of evolutionary medicine. Oxford University Press, 2009.
5. Gluckman PD, Hanson MA. Evolution, development and timing of puberty. Trends Endocrinol Metab2006;17:7-12.
6. Nesse RM, Bergstrom CT, Ellison PT, Flier JS, Gluckman PD, Govindaraju DR, et al. Evolution in health and medicine Sackler colloquium: making evolutionary biology a basic science for medicine. Proc Natl Acad Sci USA2010;107:1800-7.
7. Alonso A, Zaidi T, Novak M, Grundke-Iqbal I, Iqbal K (June 2001). "Hyperphosphorylation induces self-assembly of tau into tangles of paired helical filaments/straight filaments". Proc. Natl. Acad. Sci. U.S.A. 98 (12): 6923–8. doi:10.1073/pnas.121119298. PMC 34454. PMID 11381127.
8. Dennis J. Selkoe (2003). "Folding proteins in fatal ways". Nature 426 (6968): 900–904. doi:10.1038/nature02264. PMID 14685251.
9. Alberts, Bruce, Dennis Bray, Karen Hopkin, Alexander Johnson, Julian Lewis, Martin Raff, Keith Roberts, and Peter Walter. "Protein Structure and Function." Essential Cell Biology. Edition 3. New York: Garland Science, Taylor and Francis Group, LLC, 2010. Pg 120-170.
10. http://evolutionarypsychiatry.blogspot.com/2011_06_01_archive.html
11. http://evolutionarypsychiatry.blogspot.com/2011/06/nutrition-and-alzheimers-disease.html
12. J Amer Geriatric Soc. 2010 Mar;58(3):487-92. Metabolic syndrome and risk of dementia in older adults
13. http://diss.kib.ki.se/2005/91-7140-514-3/thesis.pdf
14. http://online.wsj.com/article/SB10001424052702303661904576452243498496516.html?mod=rss_Health

Chapter Twelve

THE MONSTER LEPTIN RESET THREAD AT MARK'S DAILY APPLE

THE VIRTUAL PATIENTS OF THE NEW PARADIGM

by Colleen Coble

This chapter is a story of five people I have never met beyond the Internet, email, or phone. They all successfully used evolutionary medicine for different medical problems. This gives you a glimpse into how regular people implement the Epi-paleo Rx. In this chapter you will meet Colleen Coble, an established fiction author, who tells her story and the story of others of tapping into the Epi-paleo Rx. You will meet Jonathon, who began his journey at 506 pounds and now is closing in on 350 pounds. You will meet a young mother, Ivy, who successfully got back into a bikini after a difficult medical history and three children. You will meet Gretchen, who overcame more than most face, and blasted herself out of a serious PCOS plateau and on to rock star status. And finally, you will meet Dexter. Dexter proves that changing your thoughts might not only change your DNA, but also may extend your life through better health. This chapter is their stories.

COLLEEN

I'm a storyteller by profession so I am used to immersing the reader in a character's challenges and trials. But the following stories are real people whose lives have been changed by Dr. Kruse's principles. I should know because I'm one of them. We have found a real community on our Mark's

Daily Apple thread and on Dr. Kruse's blog, where we discuss our own journeys and offer help to those searching for an answer.

I have struggled with my weight all of my life. I was chubby at 10, lost my first ovary at 14, then babied the second ovary along until I was 23, when I had a complete hysterectomy after the birth of our second child. That's when the pounds really began to pile on. Nothing I did changed things. When you live with obesity, it's a constant source of pain. I would look at other women who were slim and wonder what it would be like to feel normal. To be able to walk into a store and wear something in a size that wasn't a plus. I was only in my 30s, but I felt like I was 80. I tried every diet known to man, but nothing worked. But worse than the weight gain were the health issues that came with it: nearly daily migraines, fibromyalgia, celiac disease, multiple food allergies, brain fog, joint aches, and many other smaller issues that I know now were all interrelated. When my children were small, I often spent days in bed in pain and vomiting from the migraines. The headaches went from two a week, each lasting three days, to daily, debilitating pain. I had a great husband, two wonderful children, an active life, but no way out of the pit of pain and despair. I lived on pain meds and triptan drugs. My primary occupation was making sure I knew where my Imitrex was at all times. My first thought in the morning was whether my head hurt. If it didn't, I thanked God, but I knew the next migraine was lurking around the corner.

However, I've always been a can-do person, and I was determined to find an answer. I know more about migraines than most doctors because of all the research I've done looking for an answer. I realized the only person who could change my life was me. No one knows my body as well as I do. I felt if I listened to my body and studied the research, I would find an answer to my pain. If I had known how long that search would last, I might have given up. The answer to my migraine pain was one of the last pieces of my health journey.

The first piece of my personal puzzle came after finding a doctor who corrected an underlying candida problem and food allergies. I got on thyroid medication and the fibromyalgia improved. But I still wasn't well, and the weight gain didn't stop. In fact, it only intensified with the years and the migraines got even worse. I read about the link between migraines and a patent foramen ovale (PFO) heart problem, a hole in the heart that doesn't close the way it should after birth, and had a test run. Sure enough,

I had one. I was ready to get an experimental stent put in to correct it, but just in time, I read a book titled The Migraine Cure by Dr. Sergey Dzugan. When I read it, I knew it was the answer to my migraines. I have a terrific primary care doctor, and he agreed to let me try bioidentical hormones. The headaches got worse, but it was confirmation that I was on the right track. In spite of the cost, I got on the Dzugan protocol of bioidentical hormones and supplements and my migraines became a thing of the past. Relief! It was indescribable. Anyone who has suffered with constant, chronic pain understands.

But still my weight didn't budge. About three years ago I found the hCG protocol, which was another major piece of my puzzle. I lost 75 pounds, dropping from a size 20 to an eight. An eight! I could finally walk into a regular store and purchase something like the women I'd envied for years. Joy! I can't even begin to tell you how amazing that has been for me. I was willing to take on the battle with carbs to stay this size. I thought that would be my life and I was willing to pay that price.

But I was about to find another piece I'd been missing. In July of 2011 another member of the hCG forum posted a link to Dr. Kruse's blog article, Hormones 101. When I read that blog, it was like reading about my life and my health challenges. Something clicked and I just knew everything he was saying was true. This was the underlying reason for everything I'd dealt with since I was a child. I had corrected some things but not the base cause. I started the leptin reset. I didn't miss the grains or sugar since I have celiac disease and avoid gluten anyway. Besides, I had been on a low-carb diet for years, so I was used to no grains and no sugar. On the leptin reset I was never hungry and maintaining my weight became so easy. After a few weeks I was able to eat more carbohydrates (in the form of vegetables and fruit) than I had been able to eat in 30 years and still maintain my weight. Sleep became deeper. I had more energy. My hair began to grow thicker. My skin became smoother and more supple, and the age spots began to fade.

After six months of eating this way, I had labs done to see if anything had changed. Even with all the past improvements before starting the leptin reset, my cholesterol had been in the toilet at 130 total. My C-reactive protein and homocysteine levels had remained high. However, my new lab results were amazing! My C-reactive protein was .1! My homocysteine level had come down to 9 from a high of 17. And my cholesterol was 200 with my HDL at 70! 70, even for this couch potato novelist! Now I had enough cholesterol for my body to make some hormones on its own.

It is all thanks to the truths Dr. Kruse has taught me. I tell everyone about Dr. Kruse and his life-altering protocol! Not everyone listens, and I've had to come to the realization that not everyone is ready to change. Sometimes people are so used to operating with pain they can't imagine living differently. Those who are ready to hear will. I hope you are one of those.

Now I'd like to introduce you to some of my friends. I'm going to start with Jonathan. He has been an inspiration to me and to many others on the hCG forum. His determination and encouragement to others on their journeys make him a star to many of us.

JONATHAN

Jonathan took the scale out of the box and placed it on the floor. He made no move to step onto it. His pants bulged, and his belt barely fastened, so he didn't need a new scale to tell him he'd gained weight. But he'd faced every challenge thrown his way, and he wasn't going to shirk this one. He took a deep breath and stepped onto the scale. The display blinked, then settled at a number he'd never dreamed could appear: 506.

He'd tried everything to stop the upward march of his weight, so what did knowing the truth gain him? He stared at the horrendous number and vowed he would find a way. Somehow he would discover the key to his uncontrollable weight gain.

Jonathan's mother hated him. Both his mother and his grandmother beat him regularly, starting when he was about 18 months old. He developed epilepsy at that time due to head trauma. Beatings were received either standing in front of the refrigerator or tied to the bed while he was whipped with forsythia and rose bushes, when they were in season, or electrical cords and wet leather belts.

He gained a pound a month and weighed 125 by the time he was 10. His weight was a major source of pain for him. Nothing worked to slow his gains, and he suffered with sleep apnea and depression, and often thought about suicide. By the time he was 12, he took charge of the situation himself. He tried fasting until his parents put a stop to it. He forced his body into extreme forms of exercise to try to balance the mental suffering, but still his weight climbed. He was kicked out of the house at 17 and barely existed on what food he could afford to buy. He became a vegan out of necessity since he could only afford pasta and a few vegetables.

When his best friend died, he was so lonely he decided to marry his friend's sister. To his horror, he discovered he'd married a woman just like his mother. Jonathan slept in the car many nights to get away from her, while his weight and health continued to be a problem. By age 26, he weighed 365 pounds as measured on a truck scale. He followed an 800-calorie diet he found, and managed to lose 40 pounds before it stopped working for him.

His work took him to Nashville for eight months. At the same time, his doctor put him on Androgel for low testosterone, and his weight ballooned 90 pounds. He corrected the dose but still wasn't able to lose that weight. He realized that the old calories in/calories out model simply didn't work. If he ate 500 calories he didn't lose and if he ate 10,000 calories his weight didn't go up. Calorie counting was useless. His girlfriend talked him into a seeing a naturopath, and he finally began to turn his life around after agreeing to neurocranial restructuring, a procedure that involves manipulating the skull in order to provide health benefits. His health began to improve, and he returned home to find he tipped the scales at 506.

Jonathan discovered the hCG protocol at his highest weight. He lost over 100 pounds on the hCG diet but he still wasn't well. His obesity wasn't cured. He first heard of Dr. Kruse on the hCG forum. Jonathan read The Quilt, but instead of being encouraged, fresh despair gripped him: had his mother's abuse destroyed his leptin pathways? It was possible, according to Dr. Kruse. The thought of living his life this way brought fresh pain and rage at his mother. But Dr. Kruse took note of him and suggested he try a ketogenic Paleolithic diet while maintaining the rules regarding meal timing and food intake. Fat doesn't spike insulin levels, so it can be very helpful. He started on the recommended supplements and immediately began to see changes, such as better sleep, a rise in testosterone, a change in body composition, and more strength and stamina. He has been focusing on hormonal balance and thyroid correction, too. Jonathon's weight is now down to 361 pounds. His labs have improved as well.

Jonathan's biggest change, however, is he now has the key to his optimal self in his possession-his new way of thinking about how to get himself well with the Epi-paleo Rx.

Jonathan says: "There have been mental changes as well as emotional ones. Depression, which was manageable before, is really gone. I do not dwell on past issues in the slightest. My emotional demeanor is enhanced. I tend to have more good days than bad. Bad days end when my eyes close more often than not, very rarely do things last a second day. I also think more about how to get what I need from food. The Leptin Reset has drilled into my brain some things that I had begun to suspect while using hCG, and then started to be convinced of after reading The Primal Blueprint. There is not a lot of food available in the market place. Eating a ketogenic diet gives me a unique perspective. I know when protein is grain fed versus grass fed. I can tell from the way the meat tastes and especially how the fat reacts to heat. If the animal fat doesn't solidify at room temp after cooking, it is damaged. I have moved to canned salmon rather than any meat at the grocery store. I am extremely grateful that I am at a place where I can feed myself. This is never taken for granted. Eating real food is not easy in this day and time.

I feel that my story is really just starting and that in five years or so I will be proud of the story, but I am a hard case, a hard ass. Nothing short of my ideal body is going to impress me."

IVY

The crash woke her. Ivy struggled to sit up on the sofa and rubbed her eyes. The baby was crying, and the other children were supposed to be watching television, but judging by the debris on the floor, they'd helped themselves to a snack as well. How long had she been asleep? She glanced at the clock. Two hours. What was wrong with her? Life wasn't supposed to be a round of fatigue and depression.

Born in Norway, Ivy was of Indian descent but had always been fed a diet of fruit, veggies, fish, poultry, and potatoes, along with the usual additions of "healthy" grains, such as mountains of rice, pasta, and couscous. Ice cream was a daily part of her diet, and by age 10, she drank soft drinks daily. She was off and on penicillin for ear and throat infections for most of her life. When she was 23, she moved to Australia for school, where she partied and drank her way through three years of university training. She also decided to become a vegetarian She had colds, thrush and infections all the time, but didn't link her diet to the illnesses.

She lost and gained the same 25 pounds over and over again. Trapped in a cycle of binging and starvation diets, she also battled candida, gluten sensitivity, and lactose intolerance. Starting in September of 2009, she lost

35 pounds on a low-carb, low-fat diet. She ate six small meals a day, and there was no emphasis on nutritional deficiencies or the ratio of omega 3 to omega 6. In spite of the weight loss, she still struggled with dizziness, fatigue, and irritability.

After conceiving her third child, it seemed the hormonal floodgates opened. All she wanted was the thing she had denied herself: refined carbohydrates, fats, and sugar. When her daughter was born, Ivy weighed 190. She was overweight, depressed, fatigued, and lost. She felt hopeless as she napped on the sofa for hours after a sugar crash every afternoon. She felt hungrier than ever, but all the cereal, toast, pasta and rice didn't fill the hole in her belly.

Three months later she developed burning upper abdominal pain every day after breakfast. She ignored it for six weeks before seeing a doctor and being diagnosed with: nothing. The doctor admitted there might be a chance it was a food allergy, but she realized she couldn't count on a doctor for help. She was broken, and no one could start the journey to health for her. She had to take charge of this herself.

She still counts it a miracle the day she stumbled across a comment mentioning Mark's Daily Apple. After popping in to have a look, she didn't stop reading for weeks. First she read all of Mark's articles, then she moved on to the forum, where she learned her gut pain and many other health issues were due to leaky gut. She started a primal diet, began healing her gut, and felt amazing. Was this what health felt like? Then she found found Dr. Jack Kruse's blog...where she promptly felt lost. Dr. Kruse used terminology she'd never heard. But one blog turned it around for her: Why is Oprah Still Fat? Leptin 3. She understood she was leptin resistant, mineral deficient, and probably always had been.

Her body immediately responded to the big protein breakfast. There were no big changes, but the small things she'd been told to look for began to appear: heat in her body, sweating 20 minutes after meals, an increase in sex drive, and a strong desire to move. Most astounding of all, she never felt hunger. She could go seven to eight hours before she began to think about another meal. It took Ivy six weeks to begin to get the signs of leptin sensitivy, but she considers that an incredibly short time after a lifetime of damage.

Seven months later, Ivy has lost 46 pounds of fat. She sleeps soundly. She doesn't sleep on the sofa any longer but instead has the energy to play with her children. The apathy in the eyes of her friends and family compels her to share Mark's Daily Apple and Dr. Kruse's sites with them, but many tell her it's too hard. How is anything too hard when it brings about such life-changing results?

Ivy says this: "Somewhere along the line, this journey stopped being about weight loss for me. I'm searching for health and longevity, happiness and energy. I've been trapped in a hole for too long, and only recently did I get out. And it sure is beautiful out here."

GRETCHEN

Gretchen stared at the piece of paper in her hand. The words "medically discharged" wavered in her vision, and she wheezed through airways constricted by asthma. Her head was pounding, and her heart fluttered faster than the pulses of pain in her head. It was the end of her military career. Even though she'd known it was coming, seeing it in black and white made her want to sink to the floor and bury her head in her hands.

In 1999, the Air Force discharged Gretchen because of uncontrollable asthma and constant migraines. She was processed out of the military and into the VA medical system, where she was diagnosed with post-traumatic stress disorder (PTSD) and bipolar disorder. The doctors put her on a battery of drugs for her conditions, and she promptly gained 30 pounds. Her life was stressful due to continual pain and her high-pressure job as a logistics consultant for a government contractor (she was an active participant in the 9/11 response.) She battled insomnia and weight gain and joined Weight Watchers, but was never able to drop below 160 pounds.

In 2002, the VA diagnosed her with fibromyalgia and chronic fatigue syndrome. In 2004, she began to have reactions to the medications she was on, and the VA neurologist took her off her medications and sent her to a chiropractor. She found some relief from her symptoms by going gluten and dairy free, but her weight stubbornly refused to move. In fact, it began to climb again as she started her family. Six months after the birth of her second child, she was still wearing maternity clothing and was miserable at 190 pounds.

In October 2010, she stumbled upon Mark's Daily Apple. She bought The Primal Blueprint and jumped into the program. Going 100-percent grain free was easy. The hard part was kicking the sugar from her diet, which took her four months. By February 2011, she was out of maternity clothes, and in size 12 pants. Then her weight stalled again. Counting calories didn't work. Adding fats and proteins didn't work. Low-carb didn't work. No results in weight or body composition resulted from those changes.

In May 2011, she discovered Dr. Kruse's Leptin Reset thread on Mark's Daily Apple. With her usual commitment, she plunged into following the reset eating, though she continued to run and walk daily and lift weights two to three days a week, which she now thinks held her back.

Within six weeks, she began to see signs of leptin sensitivity. Her nails began growing at a phenomenal rate and she also saw an increase in her sex drive. Her cycle returned and she began sweating within the first five minutes of working out. But she also began to gain weight. Dr. Kruse told her that she had hormonal issues that she needed to test, but she balked at spending the money. Another 12 weeks went by before she finally gave in and had some labs run. She paid for most of the tests out of her flexible spending account, and they pinpointed the problem-her cortisol levels were backwards, with the main elevation occurring at night. She was dealing with pregnenolone steal syndrome, and her brain had turned off the hypothalamus-pituitary axis, essentially shutting down her thyroid to a maintenance level. She focused on fixing the cortisol through the use of adaptogens. She gave up her beloved coffee for decaf, and stopped working out.

Six weeks later, she stepped on the scale found she was 10 pounds lighter-160 pounds. She started lifting heavy things, and incorporated high intensity interval training (HIIT). She still had size 10 clothes in her closets that didn't fit. Following the leptin reset principles, and working out right before or right after dinner, made the world of difference. By December she was in size 10 suits and size eight pants and jeans.

She stepped up her efforts and focused on the circadian rhythms Dr. Kruse kept blogging about. She quit wearing sunglasses and found herself missing lunch because she wasn't hungry.

Gretchen says this: "I've seen major body composition changes since the beginning of December, as well as increases in strength with the BodyRock.tv workouts I've been doing. While I'm not optimal yet, I'm on my way. With every blog Dr. Kruse writes, another piece of my health puzzle falls into place. I'm not in a bikini yet, but I will be and I'll have a crazy six-pack of abs to complement the bikini. The most amazing thing about the entire reset is how my perspective has changed. My entire way of thinking has changed. Stress doesn't affect me like it used to. I'm a better mother and wife. Do I have bad days? Yeah, sure I do, but more often those aren't bad days but a bad moment within a day that is quickly replaced by something positive. Am I the best person I could be every day? Probably not, but that's a piece of what becoming optimal is about. Every day I'm better than I was the day before in everything: my health, my mental state, my role as a wife, my role as a mother, and my role as an employee. Yeah, the weight loss, and increased health are excellent benefits too, but each day I become a better version of me, and that for me that's the most amazing thing about what the thread has done for me."

DEXTER

Dexter hosed off the motorhome, filthy from the trip home from Alaska. He felt breathless and paused to let his belt out a little. Maybe he'd just take it off. He'd never thought he would develop what he called "Dunlap Disease." His belly had done lapped over his belt buckle. And he was 64. If he didn't change things, he was headed for an early grave.

Dexter and his wife had moved to a retirement community in Arizona with high hopes of many active years. After that trip to Alaska, he knew things would have to change if he expected to enjoy his retirement. In his youth, he'd been a pretty good softball player, so he joined a team in the community. And promptly found his stellar throwing arm had deteriorated into a pathetic remnant of its former self. He was the weak link for his team instead of being the asset he'd hoped. So he signed up with a personal trainer for strength training. The first thing he received was a nutritional guideline that said to limit his diet to 75 grams of carbohydrates a day. He had only a vague concept of carbs, but he was determined to do this thing right. At 62 and a body fat of 36 percent, he knew he had his work cut out for him. At the end of three months, he had dropped 25 pounds and decreased his body fat to 25 percent.

Encouraged by this success, he purchased the P90X DVD exercise program. He dropped another 20 pounds and his body fat fell to 20 percent. But he was so sore that he couldn't function well. So he started to research what made people fat. He read Dr. Michael Eades' Protein Power. Then he found the Gary Taubes book Good Calories, Bad Calories, then others on exercise, such as Dr. Doug McGuff's Body By Science. He started lifting to failure with very heavy weights.

About this time, he discovered Paleohacks.com and became an avid participant there. There was another poster on Paleohacks whose handle was "The Quilt," now known to many in the Paleo and primal world as Dr. Jack Kruse.

Dexter found the doctor's postings to be very cryptic. Dr. Kruse appeared to want the readers to ferret out exactly what he was trying to say and to discover the pearls he was posting on their own. But the more Dexter read, the more the doctor made sense. When he read Dr. Kruse's ideas about how our thoughts can change DNA, he realized that he could change his health by his food choices. Sugary sodas or wheat-laden pancakes with syrup were incredibly harmful to his body, so he cut them out.

The Quilt and the "Monster" thread at Mark's Daily Apple provided Dexter's first real guide for his journey toward healthy living. He found it easy to eat 50 grams of protein within 30 minutes of rising in the morning. He loved the coconut oil and other good fats that he was encouraged to add to his diet. The fog he lived with lifted almost immediately. He took the information to his primary care physician, who ordered tests and a sleep study. Dexter discovered he had sleep apnea, even though he was at 12 percent body fat and a healthy weight of 160. His CPAP machine will arrive soon.

Dexter says this: "Many folks think I am whacked out because what I have to say is so totally different from what the mainstream medical profession preaches. My response is this, just try it for 30 days and see how you feel. Works every time if the person will follow my advice for 30 days. This is what is called assisting others to overcome their health challenges without expecting any reward other than satisfaction of helping a fellow human with their health challenges. Paying it forward to others what Dr. Kruse has given to us."

Dexter just summed up what all of us feel. We are out to change the world with radical ideas that actually work. We want to help others achieve the same benefits we've found. And we want to say thank you to Dr. Kruse. Thank you for giving us the tools to fix ourselves. Thank you for being so generous with your time. And thank you for being bold enough to swim against the tide.

Chapter Thirteen

PROOF THAT THE EPI-PALEO RX IS THE PALEOLITHIC DIET OF ALL TIME

MY MUSIC CITY MIRACLE OF JANUARY 9, 2012

Physicians and research scientists collect and analyze information to develop treatments or to gain new insights through experimentation. The problem is we usually think about this information reductively instead of connecting the dots. This chapter shows you how the Epi-paleo Rx might help you change the way you think about your built-in owner's manual.

These are bits of scientific information that I knew about in 2005, but I had no idea then how they all fit together. This chapter is how I found order in this chaos and used it to change my own life, my family's life, and those of my patients since 2008.

Knowledge only occurs when we tie the bits together with a plausible theory. I realized in 2007 that leptin might do more than just regulate getting fat or thin. I thought leptin might hold the key to all Neolithic diseases and lead us to our ultimate longevity. I told you how I used the Leptin Rx reset protocol to help people lose weight, but I decided to test another hypothesis that sprang from my own weight loss journey and the chronic pain I had in my surgically repaired knee. This chapter chronicles how I tapped the Epi-paleo Rx to improve my former self. The bits of information I listed above came together in my mind during the last 35 years and culminated in my taking the biggest risk of my life to prove a thought experiment. I took this challenge head-on because of the challenge Wahls accepted as she fought for her life against multiple sclerosis. It really motivated me to do something aggressive that might make a difference for others.

In 2009, I began to really think about the constant knee pain I had after my surgery, and how I could use what I had learned to help people. It became clear to me the information could apply to my neurosurgery patients as well. In the Leptin Rx chapter, I told you how I figured out how to cure my own obesity. It was pretty straightforward, requiring no drugs or surgery and no special testing outside of blood work. In my first podcast with Jimmy Moore in May of 2011, I explained how I held off on my own knee surgery until my inflammatory markers lowered. What I did not tell listeners is that I started off with an HS-CRP over three. This is high and showed I still had some leptin issues left. When I had my surgery my level was around one. The surgery went well, but for one year after I had a constant and nagging discomfort in my knee. I complained often but did little about it. Then something happened that opened my eyes. As I continued to test my blood, I saw my HS-CRP fall to 0.001 and my vitamin D rise to 70 ng/mL. Simultaneously, my knee pain went away completely overnight. I was able to run and deadlift and had experienced an amazing change overall a year after the surgery. I was also very fit and weighed around 200 pounds. If you remember back to the Leptin Rx chapter, I had a blast of insight at the foot of Michelangelo's David. Well, I had another one the day my knee pain went away for good. I wondered if becoming extremely leptin sensitive could help my spine patients recover from surgery without much pain or hospitalization.

So I began to do some research and met two women on a spine health forum who both suffered from chronic spondylotic myelopathy with severe chronic pain. This is a neck problem that results in compression of the spinal cord and lifelong chronic pain. It is a miserable outcome from an injury or a surgery. I made friends with both of them and learned about their cases in detail. Neither one lived in my city and I still have never met them to this day. After talking with them for months, I realized both ladies were leptin resistant and eating a SAD. I began to wonder if their diet was behind their chronic pain? So I began to see how a ketogenic Paleolithic diet would affect chronic pain in my own patients. I also put them on a combination of fish oil and krill oil to lower inflammation, and followed their inflammatory markers and vitamin D levels. What I found after doing this with just a few patients shocked me. I was able to perform large spine operations on these patients and I did not have to use as many narcotics post-operative as usual. The bigger finding was that I was able to send them home earlier with less rehabilitation. In some cases, I became so bold that I did less invasive surgeries than I was used to doing, and I found these patients did even better! When I changed their diet and added some supplements, their surgical outcomes were dramatically better.

I decided to do a thought experiment based upon these findings. I wondered if I could predict outcomes based on their blood tests and hormone status. I began to do this constantly and found not one patient had a normal vitamin D level in the first three years I tested people. Their HS-CRP was also usually quite elevated, and most had underlying hormonal issues tied to their inflammation. I went back and did some more reading on the neuroendocrine response in surgery and decided it was time to see if it was possible to reduce pain completely without surgery. I soon found my usage of epidural steroids and narcotics dropped 85 percent the first year just by altering patients' diets. I stopped routinely placing pedicle screws in the lower back (for spinal fusions), because I found I no longer need to when I treated patients' inflammatory conditions first. They also began to lose weight. A lot of weight, like I did. I discussed this with three physicians in my hospital and told them I thought I was on to something pretty big. My competitors were kind of shocked that I stopped doing big cases in 2007 that normally made us surgeons good money. They were perplexed at what I was doing, and they often made derogatory comments around the hospital about it because they just could not fathom it.

The funny thing was my patients were getting better quicker with smaller surgeries. Word around town started to spread, and soon I began seeing more difficult cases-patients with serious chronic pain. Many of them also improved dramatically. It was at this point that my practice evolved. I stopped doing conventional spine surgery and began to incorporate what I had learned. I practiced medicine using an evolutionary prism from that day forward. Many of my patients' diseases improved as I treated their back and neck pain. Their lipids improved, normal hair growth returned to their extremities, calcium build up in their arteries resolved, dental health improved, and libido that had been absent for decades returned. It was quite remarkable really! Fragile bones were restored to health, heart disease reversed, and I cured some type 2 diabetics without even trying. It was pretty cool, honestly.

Then something fortuitous happened. It was September 2007 and I was watching a football game. Buffalo Bills tight end Kevin Everett fell to the turf paralyzed after a hit. The surgeon infused Everett's body with ice-cold saline and Everett went on to make a miraculous recovery in a few weeks. Later that year, many in the spine surgery literature claimed his recovery was due to the fact that it was not a complete spinal cord injury, not the novel use of hypothermia. Many did not believe the cold had much to do with his recovery. Everett was interviewed on TV later that year and mentioned something casually to the interviewer that caught my attention. He said the pain from his surgery while intubated was not too bad either! His surgeon had told him it might be a painful operation in areas where he could feel, but he said that wasn't the case. Moreover, since he recovered so quickly, he reported very little pain even when he regained all his neurologic function. I had done the same surgery many times and I knew it was a painful operation. The incongruity intrigued me, given the unusual circumstances of his case. So I went looking for why this occurred.

I uncovered data on children with frostbite injuries that shocked me, yet fit with Everett's claims. These studies reported the children become insensitive to pain before they developed painful nerve paresthesias, due to the length of time they were exposed to the cold. They also mentioned something else that piqued my interest. It was difficult to surgically reconstruct their faces because the cold had significantly and permanently atrophied the fat of the exposed areas.

The articles reported that the fat cells vanished permanently! Popsicle panniculitis is a dermatologic condition in which exposure to low temperatures can selectively damage subcutaneous fat while leaving skin completely intact. Well, since a lot of my own fat cells vanished too, I had to look deeper. I found plastic surgeons were developing a tool to remove fat without surgery called the "Zeltiq procedure." Dieter Manstein and R. Rox Anderson at The Wellman Center at Massachusetts General Hospital originated the concept. They developed it further in a number of experiments on pigs and reported their data in 2008. Plastic surgeons began used freezing cold metal plates on patients' body parts to melt fat away without surgery! It appears that fatty tissue cooled below body temperature but above freezing temperature undergoes localized cell death followed by an "unusual local inflammatory response." This was a stunning to me because they had no idea how this process worked biochemically. I felt immediately

I knew how it might work. It had to be tied to leptin function at some level. I kept reading and found that some of the people complained they were left completely numb in this area of treatment and insensate to pain for quite some time. This data also fit with Everett's story of his own surgery. These links made me look deeper for a biological reason. I began to wonder if I could somehow use temperature to eliminate pain in surgery or for chronic pain patients? After all, I was a neurosurgeon, and on my business card it says, "my goal is to keep you free of pain and discomfort." What I could not reconcile was why cold temperatures caused permanent fat atrophy. I went back to the library to investigate this link and wondered if it was tied to leptin function at all. The library turned up nothing, but a TV program opened my eyes.

I was watching a Discovery Channel program about astronauts training in pools of icy cold water. The narrator mentioned NASA's studies of Sherpas, the porters who guide people up Mount Everest, showed they lose unbelievable amounts of weight because of the cold temperatures. I was stunned again. Here was another link between fat and cold. The narrator went on to say NASA astronauts also lost weight on space walks because of the deep freeze of space, and they had to make suits to offset these losses. They used the ice-cold pools to train astronauts how to tolerate the weight loss and other physiologic changes as they worked. He did not go into detail so I scoured NASA's websites and space literature to learn more but did not find much. I did learn, however, that NASA shared this data with the U.S. Olympic Swim Team, which uses the same techniques to make their athletes trimmer and faster. I found a lot of information on training sites for Olympic swimmers that training in 50-degree water allows them to do some amazing things. They are able to train longer while eating more and still not gain any weight. In fact, most of them leaned out considerably no matter what they ate. I learned the colder it was, the more weight one would lose, the more one could eat and not gain weight, and that cold destroyed appetite. The swimmers also mentioned the cold water often made their skin numb, which made training in the water easier. It appears a cold environment makes one less sensitive to pain, with the effect lasting long after the cold exposure. I knew this had to be linked to leptin function in some way.

During this time, I was reading about frontier physicians and the Inuit in the Arctic Circle. I read an account from the famous Albert Schweitzer in 1913 that the Inuit were very healthy and had no evidence of heart disease or cancer. They were also trim and muscular, and ate a diet of raw marine animals loaded with fat and protein. Schweitzer also mentioned they could brave the cold wind and freezing water for tremendously long times while hunting, seemingly impervious to the cold's effects that were so painful to him.

These discoveries led me to read about "Milankovitch theories" from the World War I era. Miluntin Milankovitch was a civil engineer and mathematician who theorized variations in the earth's eccentricity, axial tilt, and orbit determined climatic patterns through a process called orbital forcing. His work showed there were longer, rhythmic cycles in the earth's history based upon the mathematics of our orbit. At the time, I was sure evolution was connected to these cycles, so I looked in depth at vitamin D data as tied to our climate. I found D3 is made in the skin when 7-dehydrocholesterol reacts with ultraviolet light (UVB) at wavelengths between 270 and 300 nm in humans. I knew that peak synthesis of vitamin D occurred in humans between 295 and 297 nm wavelengths of sunlight. These wavelengths are present in sunlight when the UV index is greater than three. I found that a UV index greater than 3 occurs daily within the tropics, daily during the spring and summer seasons in temperate regions, and almost never within the polar circles. I also found that latitude does not consistently predict the average serum vitamin D level of a population. This was a big clue that evolution accounted for electrons from food another way.

In reading about these phenomena something else occurred to me. Most of the earth's snow and ice lies at high latitudes. Because of this, and using Milankovitch's theories, one could postulate that any lowered tilt in the earth's axis favored the formation of ice ages. The two major reasons for this belief are a reduction in overall summertime solar radiation, and the additional reduction in mean solar radiation at high latitudes. This was technical science to be sure, and I did not know what to make of it at the time, but intuitively it seemed important so I wrote it down. I continued to read about these cycles and read a report on computer modeling I found interesting, too. The scientists used computer models to study more extreme tilts of our axis than those that have occurred in the Earth's history. They hypothesized climate extremes at high obliquity, or a more sharply angled tilt, would be particularly threatening to advanced life forms. Mother Nature has to be paying attention to a risk this dire. They also reported that high obliquity would not likely sterilize the Earth totally, but it would make it more difficult for a "fragile, warm-blooded, land-based life" to thrive as it does today.

Mountain climbers succumb to acute elevation sickness over the height of 8,000 feet due to low oxygen and extreme cold. It would take someone close to a month to acclimate to Mount Everest's altitude at base camp before a climb. Not acclimating correctly can cause cerebral or pulmonary edema and death. It takes Sherpas only a week since they are adapted to the environment.

Being too cold is not optimal-there is a limit to how cold temperature can be used by humans and evolution. I found some more data that lowering our skin temp to 50-55 degrees is the sweet spot for fat loss and pain control.

I know from my patients who were NFL players that cold tubs were quite popular after games to recover from injuries, but I could not fathom how they tolerated it. Most of them told me they did not have to be in the tub very long for relief. This was the same thing I discovered about cold in other areas of science. If we can adapt to a colder temperature, we can use it to help us do some interesting things we might not otherwise be able to, and this extends far past the exposure.

I then began testing in my hot tub by putting 40 pounds of ice on my chest and belly while my legs and torso were submersed in the 100 degree water. It was tolerable for 10 minutes. I kept doing it regularly until I could tolerate 45 minutes, and I checked my skin temperature with probes from our anesthesia. It got down to 50 degrees. I was also completely numb for almost five days! I noticed the longer I went, the more numb I got. My skin became intensely red during the sessions as well. At this point I became bold. I began to take ice baths in the bathroom tub with 60-80 pounds of ice and managed to stay in the tub for up to six hours at times. I even mentioned this to a physician in town and she thought I was nuts. One night I even fell asleep in the tub for close to 10 hours. After this, I found for close to two weeks that I had no hunger and the areas that had been covered by the icy water areas were numb.

All this was interesting from a clinical standpoint and I felt it was time to try this on some patients. The problem was patients weren't willing to soak in ice baths, so I compromised. I started using cooling blankets on them, but the blankets never got cold enough to really work. They are designed to get one's temperature down to 96-98 from a normal fever. Nevertheless, their requirements for narcotics dropped significantly, even with such a small temperature difference. One of these patients gave me a book by John Sarno on meditation and the treatment of low back pain, which he said had really helped him. I read the book and added meditation to the cold experiments I did in my hot tub. I even posted some of the pictures on Facebook and my friends thought I was nuts. I found the combination of meditation and cold was remarkable for numbing areas of my body. I was then able to make certain parts of my body numb for a few seconds just with thoughts. The cold in combination with the meditation worked much better. I really wanted to try this on a surgery patient but I did not have the opportunity to cut on someone and not give them pain medication.

After reading Sarno's book, I went back to the library to see if leptin function and temperature might be linked to pain control. I learned the reason the Inuit might be so cold adapted is that ice ages occurred much faster than we had previously thought, something researchers discovered using carbon-14 dating on core ice samples from the Arctic and Antarctica. I also learned about sub-arctic amphibians who made themselves diabetic on purpose to withstand the freezing. This was another evolutionary link to the puzzle. I had known from other readings that diabetes is actually protective in some cases, something biology still uses it at times as a tool. Higher glucose levels in the frog's blood acts as an antifreeze, an evolutionary adaptation. This link really made me think deeper.

The Inuit lived in chronically cold and dark climates, exposed to freezing wind and water as they hunted and fished. The polar seas have the highest nutrient-dense food chains and the highest levels of DHA on the planet, which explains why the Inuit were so fit and rugged and adapted to the cold. This is also why they appeared to be immune to heart disease and cancer, according to Schweitzer.

I also learned about life at the South Pole. I knew the climate there was far worse than the North Pole and no humans lived there normally, but emperor penguins did. They survived by forming groups to move in the dead of winter. They brooded their young in darkness, in temperatures as cold as -88 degrees Fahrenheit, in wind that blew up to 100 mph, and without eating for four months! I also learned that, like the Sherpas, the penguins lost a lot of weight without apparent appetite during this four-month ordeal. During my exploration of marine science, I also learned about the migration patterns of the great white shark. These sharks traveled huge distances across the globe, although scientists used to think they were predominately locally based predators. Scientists began to track these animals with GPS probes, finding some sharks journeyed more than 10,000 miles in less than a year! They also found they only feed in relatively temperate water, not in the warm tropical waters of the equator. They tend to eat in Australia, off the tip of Africa, and on the west coast of the United States and Mexico. When they re-caught the tagged sharks and sampled their blood, they found something even more amazing-these sharks never seem to show any signs of aging. We still do not know how long these sharks live, but we do know they have extremely low metabolic rates and can go a long time without eating. They can eat once every two months and still live a perfectly normal life. The scientists believe the sharks' diet and their cold-water environment are linked to these findings. I reread about the Inuit and Antarctic animal species and learned they were also long-lived. The same was true of Russians in Siberia and the farmers in Patagonia. Now I knew I was on to something really big. It appeared a ketogenic diet and cold temperature were somehow linked to longevity, pain control, leptin function, and low appetite.

I wondered about these links and I went back to have a look at my pictures from Florence, Italy for inspiration. I knew leptin was linked to the circadian rhythms of light and dark, but could it also be linked to geothermal temperature cycles?

EVOLUTIONARY PRISM FORMS THE CORE OF THE EPI-PALEO RX

I thought back to my childhood and the Museum of Natural History. I was a dinosaur freak as a kid. I used to go to the museum probably 75 times a year. I loved it. I distinctly remember a guide in the Hall of Evolution telling us that as time passed and more species evolved, evolutionary pressures increased, causing evolution to speed up. We are not aware of this because we do not live long to notice it. It is akin to not being able to feel the Earth rotate. Then I remembered what Einstein did in discovering the theory of relativity. He did no formal experiments because he could not go into space in 1904 to test his theories, so he used his mind to complete a thought experiment.

So I thought about why temperature and light would matter to life and evolution. Then it all clicked for me. More than 65 million years ago, the Cretaceous-Paleogene extinction event, also known as the K-T event, involved large-scale mass extinction of animal and plant species over a short period of time. It's believed an asteroid wiped out the dinosaurs. An asteroid strike many have occurred twice in earth's history, based on geologic and fossil records. The largest would be the Permo-Triassic extinction event more than 252 million years ago, which wiped out an estimated 90 percent of life. But the event I most remembered learning about growing up in New York City was the K-T event in Mexico. So I thought to myself, how might the K-T extinction play a role in our geothermal cycles, cold adaptation, and leptin? We know about 60 percent of all species below the K-T boundary are not present above the line that divides the "Age of Dinosaurs" and the "Age of Mammals." In fact, dinosaurs were not among the most numerous of the casualties according to the fossil record. The worst hit organisms were those in the oceans. It appeared that many land-based and sea-based dinosaurs were killed, except the ones who could fly.

I taught both my kids as toddlers about the one dinosaur that could fly, Archaeopteryx. This dinosaur was my favorite so I made sure both of my kids learned about it. I learned this species was the key to the evolution of the modern bird from theropod dinosaurs. Never in a million years did I think this one bit of information might be a critical link to one day figuring out what the Epi-paleo Rx for life really is.

How do we know that birds came from dinosaurs? All modern birds have the same hip articulation that dinosaur fossils show. The scientists hypothesized the earth was a ball of fire for at least a year after the asteroid's impact. But what if they were wrong about this? Nothing in the fossil or geologic record says this was totally true. I also remember learning about the "fern spiking event" in close proximity to the K-T event. A fern spike, as evidenced by an abundance of fern spores in the fossil record, usually happens immediately after an extinction event. So there was some science to saying they may not be spot on in their guess. What if the flying dinosaurs made it to the highest peaks to get away from the fire and were able to survive this ordeal? We know that mammals survived underground and came to dominate the planet in about 66 million years. We showed up about 2.5 million years ago. This rapid change in environment had to impact all life on earth especially at the poles where there were temperature extremes. Then I thought about those mammals and why they were underground to begin with.

I would imagine all animals that survived might have this DNA change in them as proof. I also recalled that they believe the asteroid hit somewhere around the Yucatan peninsula in Mexico. So I reasoned most land-based life would have been wiped out first around the Yucatan, and all the surviving species would have had to adapt to colder northern and southern climates out of necessity. This quickly would have selected for survival in the colder climates. I imagined that eventually natural selection shrunk the dinosaurs that flew to the top of these cold peaks because food was sparse. They likely would have evolved feathers for insulation from the cold and for long-distance flight to search for food.

It sounds really far fetched until you look at the present-day Arctic Snow Goose or the Arctic Tern. They both fit my theory perfectly. The geese make an annual 3,000-mile flight from the Yucatan peninsula to the Arctic Tundra. The terns make an annual 10,000-mile flight from North to South Pole. Maybe these birds where the direct descendants of the original theropod dinosaurs. Maybe our leptin receptor evolved to account for temperature because of what happened to the dinosaurs. I thought this thought experiment was "out there," but something made primal sense about it to me.

Evolution is about the survival of the fittest. Maybe evolution goes for broke in a devastation situation. Without serious deviation from the mean, true progress becomes impossible. Biology does not settle for average but shoots for ultimate survival when faced with devastation. I knew mathematics, food, and adaptation to cold had to be part of the equation. Most people are intrigued by the written work of da Vinci, Michelangelo, and Einstein, but they are not easy works to read. All three wrote in ciphers and their texts were ridiculously hard to understand, but it made scholars and scientists work harder to get the true meaning of their work. I thought maybe evolutionary biology used the reasoning they did. You might lose 90 percent of people this way, and it drives humans crazy trying to figure it out, but when those 10 percent left standing connect the dots, we reach a tipping point of understanding. I wondered if biology might use the same strategy in a cataclysmic event?

I knew from mathematics that any network becomes optimized and generates faster learning with rapid adaptation, making a tipping point occur faster than one could imagine. It is called a "Pareto distribution," or "Bradford power laws." I wondered if biology used it to ensure the survivors not only survived, but also their evolution sped up. People learn faster with complexity and ambiguity because they become more attentive to detail. Once the first few survivors get it, the rest follow by the standard power law mathematics. When I looked at how far mammals have come in a short 67 million years, it dawned on me this is how evolutionary biology made sure the animals left after the K-T event would survive. It selected for ultimate survival and did not settle. It also dawned on me evolution put this design for ultimate survival in our DNA. Ultimate survival is an epigenetic phenomenon of this biologic power law. After a few initially survive, and once the epigenetic program works, the growth of the surviving species will then be explosive. This is why evolution has sped up from primates to humans. Because of power laws, I believe the development of our Neolithic cortex outpaced the Paleolithic genes that control our biochemistry. The implications of this are vast-we are in the Dark Ages about how these mathematical laws could hurt us. Somehow, I thought, the asteroid had to be a powerful beacon for this biologic cipher.

The more northern and southern animals had to retreat for safety, and altered light made for harsher seasons. I knew the light cycle and leptin were clearly linked, and I now believe leptin is also yoked to the seasons, because life had to survive extreme climates after the K-T asteroid hit. This made sense to me but I kept it to myself, calling it "Factor X" in my mind. The Arctic was cold, and these animals had to dive for fish in frigid polar seas. I remembered reading about the Korean War veterans and frostbite studies in high school. Some reports from American soldiers serving in the Korean War and elsewhere indicate they believed dark skin was more prone to frostbite than white skin, because it emits more heat. I knew this observation was true, but not for reason they guessed. It is because dark skin makes you more insensate to cold, so you will expose yourself longer to the elements to get to food to survive! This was the Epi-paleo Rx for survival in eons past showing up in the Korean War when the harsh environment epigenetically signaled for it to be expressed.

I thought the same ecologic situations would be selected for in the oceans around Antarctica because of the same relationship with cold and light. Land-based inhabitants there could not get enough vitamin D from the sun. They were driven to acquire it from sea animals who concentrate vitamin D in their bodies because they feed on plankton in the sub-polar photic zone. It also appears the most nutrient dense part of our planet remains at the extremes when it comes to oceanic biology-90 percent of the living biome on our planet still resides in the seas, tundra, alpine environments, and polar regions of the planet.

Maybe a cold environment is what the primordial condition for life is. Consider the supporting evidence. The tropics remain a veritable waste land of marine nutrient density because of the power of the sun. Might this be a lingering effect of the K-T asteroid impact point with Earth? I knew that if something occurred on a macro level it also had to occur on a subatomic level because of the laws of quantum biology. Remember, this impact occurred 67 million years ago, and we came to be 2.5 million years ago. Using that scale, it is clear evolution has rapidly sped up. Whoever survived the K-T hit had to have the machinery to survive it programmed into their DNA by natural selection. Then, I reasoned, it must be in our own DNA today. We may not use it now, so it would not be expressed until a stimulus once again activated the survival strategy. I looked for more proof of this theory. I thought if I were right about this, then it meant the diet that worked best back then for survival had to be the best diet for today. Remember, life is about surviving by creating electrons from food. Electron exchange is what makes the world go round and keeps our leptin receptor happy. I suspect this is why life is abundant in the ocean, since our greatest food source has always been in the oceans. The survival of any animal back then required nutrient dense foods from the polar seas to provide those electrons for energy. It also follows that what is true on a functional macro level in biology has to be true on a subatomic biochemical level. So, I asked, what is the dietary blueprint to which we are best adapted?

THE FIRST-EVER EVOLUTIONARY EXPERIMENT

We evolved from the animals that had to navigate this set of circumstances. Based on my study of evolution and evolutionary medicine, it appears that every living cell carries within it billions of years of evolutionary experimentation. What happened to animals during the K-T event is hardwired into our DNA at some level, and the fact that we are alive is proof of their success. What Paleobiology tells us is that eutherian (placenta-based) mammals fared far better than metatherian (yolk sac-based/larvae form) mammals in the K-T extinction. Scientists have never figured out why this happened.

I think I might have, and it's all about leptin's evolutionary advantages. Leptin controls placental function and oocyte (egg cell) maturation in eutherian mammals, including humans. It allows for hibernation and low food consumption in cold temperatures. This is precisely why these animals survived this impact-they were hibernating, and leptin controls that ability! Mammals with placentas survived because they already had in their DNA the antidote to the extreme cold weather that occurred after the K-T event. Another more curious thing that happened at the K-T event also points to evolution's favoring of placental-based mammals. We know from fossil records that that these eutherian mammals fared better than the metatherian mammals in the northern hemisphere. But both species took a major hit in the K-T impact in the southern hemisphere. For many years this confused me until I researched the leptin link. I looked at gravity and infrared maps of the Chicxulub Crater, where it is believed the asteroid hit. The crater shows the direction of the impact was from north to south. This means the super-hot ejecta from the asteroid's impact was spewed mostly in the southern hemisphere, below the Yucatan peninsula, and that animals in the northern hemisphere had an advantage in avoiding fires. I also think the impact likely occurred in the dead of winter. Why? Because this is when mammals would have been underground hibernating, oblivious to the catastrophe occurring on the surface of the planet.

Is there any evidence for this theory? Look at a map of the crater and then look at the species who survived the event. It all fits. Even today, there is less density of life in the southern hemisphere than the northern hemisphere. Life was likely decimated in the southern hemisphere. This is why we see so many new and unusual species in Australia and New Guinea. Remember, since the K-T event, evolution has sped up. It appears to me this is why the only true permanent inhabitant of Antarctica is the emperor penguin. It also explains why we do not see many hominid skeletons in the Paleolithic fossil record. I bet there were very small numbers of hominids that rapidly appeared. The rapid increase in evolution also means that epigenetic selection also sped up. This means that further climatic changes would have made even more dramatic impacts to our genome. I think if you look at my blog from February 22, 2012 you will see this case laid out in detail.

I believe Mother Nature selected for animals with leptin receptors that can fuel energy in cold climates worldwide. This planetary event forced evolution to use "quantum biologic effects" to figure out the best way for the remaining life to survive. The remaining animals were the mammals hibernating underground! The leptin hormone and receptor are critical in the biology of all eutherian mammals. Animals before us did not use a complex leptin receptor. Mammalian leptin receptor function is quite complex and far reaching, controlling oocyte development and mammalian reproductive potential. This means it directly masters all of our epigenetic switches. And it works fast because evolutionary speed has increased. It does not take hundreds of generations to make changes now. This means more Neolithic mismatches are possible for humans today than were possible for our ancestors.

What is evolution's prime directive? Survival of the species by reproductive fitness. What did evolution do? It was pressured to sculpt the leptin receptor to create the ultimate survival plan for those animals left standing. It explains the geologic record for dinosaurs when you look at it this way. Leptin structure and homology is that big of a deal. How it adapts and rewires is based on circadian signals. Does this sound familiar to anyone who has used my Leptin Rx reset or read the blog post about how the Leptin Rx works? How about the Cold Thermogenesis blog series? The leptin receptor functions tremendously well in low light and cold temperatures. I think there are other variables, but not in mammals. (That is for another book.)

This is why mammals have placentas and all early mammals hibernated to survive the harsh tundra climates. Placental leptin function appears to be why mammals dominated the planet after the K-T impact. The surviving species then expanded much more than once believed because evolution used power laws to guarantee survival by speeding up evolution. It made evolving feathers for the flying dinosaurs an easy task. Flying dinosaurs were the only other lucky species that didn't hibernate, but they escaped extinction because they could move to higher elevations quickly by flying! I have often thought the Arctic Tern is modern version of Archaeopterx. If you Google its life cycle, you will be amazed how it fits perfectly with what I just shared.

FACTOR X EQUALS EPIGENETIC SPEED

We are the biologic remnants of that great catastrophe. The proof is in how our leptin receptor functions with respect to food. This is when leptin became the top dog on my Quilt document. It was critical to all life left on this planet after K-T and conferred huge advantages for survival. Only needing food six months out of the year and being able to brave the cold without eating or being hungry would have been a huge advantage to life post K-T. If that receptor could rewire to destroy hunger, improve energy efficiency, and decrease caloric need, survival would be guaranteed. Moreover, if I am correct it means that Factor X is buried within our DNA, and tapping it can help us solve any disease we face today.

I believed proof would be found by testing the leptin receptor's ability in extreme situations. All of life's successes are tied to effective energy metabolism. Cold thermogenesis is how this program is launched in all mammals. It guarantees ultimate survival as long as we are eating a ketogenic Paleolithic diet. Other versions of this diet are very good as well, but none can be considered optimal for health. I learned that a ketogenic version of the Paleolithic diet is the greatest adaptation for planetary extremes and confers health, leanness, control of appetite, and longevity. This is why I believe we are best adapted to eat this way. It is hardwired into our owner's manual.

I think as we moved around the planet after the K-T event, we adopted an omnivore diet because environmental pressures subsided. This altered the epigenetic expression of our DNA's capability. This is the critical factor that eventually created our brains in a warm climate. This set us up for many biologic mismatches and is the source of most Neolithic diseases we face today.

But it does not negate how powerful that diet is for our survival. Because we do not routinely see its benefit, we do not have perspective, in the way we can't perceive the Earth's rotation or evolutionary speed. However, our longevity is tied to how we eat because of our history. Evolutionary directives came up with the blueprint to shape the leptin receptor. Moreover, I realized that this information not only linked the leptin receptor to energy from food, but also extended to pain control, weight and appetite control, and maybe even longevity. This was all built into the ancient pathways. I have written extensively on this pathway on my blog. How far might FACTOR X take me? I had to continue the thought experiment.

HOW DOES NEUROSURGERY FIT IN?

I first made the link between cold and pain in the early 2000s at a medical meeting. I learned that a primary care doctor named Ritchie Shoemaker linked alpha MSH and leptin directly to pain control. Since I had made the evolutionary connections already, I had another eureka moment. I wondered if we could somehow modulate alpha MSH and inflammatory cytokines to help patients with chronic pain? I also realized it might connect with longevity, low inflammation, controlled appetite, and leptin, too. I knew I had to test this hypothesis on modern humans at some point, as the science behind it was too deep to ignore. Discovering these things made me aware of my own blind spots as a neurosurgeon, and that many of the things I believed to be true no longer were. So I decided to erase everything in my head I had been taught and examine medicine through an evolutionary prism. This produced three ideas of how I could prove this theory and test my cold thermogenesis theory. So far, the Leptin Rx is proving itself pretty well on the Internet and in my office. It is what cured me. The second and third thought experiments were radically different and bolder, but both would confirm my theory was valid. It also meant I was going to be burying lots of scientific dogma I had been taught. William Osler, the great medical doctor, said, "The eye cannot see what the mind does not know." The Leptin Rx reset was the first train stop in my thought experiment. I added cold thermogenesis to my own reset to shed fat.

The second train stop was the effect of cold thermogenesis on pain elimination in mammals so they could forage for food in deep cold. Mind you, we would not need much to get by, but we need some food. I felt cold thermogenesis had to control pain so we could enter the nutrient-dense polar seas.

Train stop three was a much bigger thought experiment. It required me to imagine what would happen to a mammalian somatic cell over 67 million years if evolution sped up, and if epigenetic control of the genome sped up even faster, allowing for the emergence of the human brain. Once that brain evolved, it had the ability to create its own environment and own realities despite the body's older Paleolithic genes. This situation required me to consider how time was relative for evolution and its epigenetic control switch, and what mismatches might happen. Then, in 2006, I got my answer to the solution. I was imagining what would happen to a cell's telomere lengths as epigenetic speed accelerated generation to generation over 67 million years from the K-T event. Telomere lengths are the ultimate arbiter of cellular fitness and survival. If a diet is optimal then it should lengthen our telomere length and not shorten it. So, I had a framework with which to try and disprove my theory.

BACK TO THE THOUGHT EXPERIMENTS

You learned about these earlier in the book when we discussed fibromyalgia and Lyme disease. Alpha-MSH is tied to the stimulation of melanocytes, which is why people who lived in polar extremes also had darker skin. Most people think "white" when they think polar extremes. Most polar wildlife is dominated by the color white, but not the major adapted inhabitants, like the Inuit in the north or the emperor penguins in the south. It was during this medical meeting that I realized why the Sherpas needed to eat lard and butter to maintain their weight as they guided people to the top of Everest. I also remembered that the Bactrian camels were the neighbors of the Sherpas in the Gobi desert, just north of Mount Everest. They lived in a cold desert eating next to nothing and three pounds of snow a day to quench their thirst. Snow never melts there because it's too cold. Camels can only eat small amounts of snow because their bodies can't handle large amounts, so they eat and drink only a small amount.

It seemed to me life had different requirements when temperature was the key factor, and that cold thermogenesis would decrease the Sherpas' inflammatory cytokines to such low levels that they would have the lowest amount of leptin and the highest amounts of adiponectin imaginable. This explained why they were dead thin, had no appetite for food, and did not need a lot of water to survive, like the people they guided up the mountain. They were the human correlates to the camels in the Gobi. It explained why they could exist on diets very low in calories compared to non-cold-adapted people. Calorie restriction was already embedded into the ancient metabolic pathway.

Extreme, rapid emptying of leptin from adipocytes also completely explained why the skin of children with frostbite became numb and they lost their fat cells as they recovered from their cold injuries. Low leptin causes fat apoptosis. The fat just shrinks. This is how mammals survive in brutal winters. It is the antidote for insulin resistance. In his talk, Shoemaker pointed out that patients with bio-toxin diseases had very low levels of alpha-MSH due to toxic exposures, which caused increased sensitivity to pain. This means that high alpha-MSH selects for pain control. So cold has to induce alpha-MSH, and it does! Things were falling into to place for me at a quick pace now and I knew I was going to have to prove it soon. The concept of safe starches and longevity were now becoming mainstream in the blogosphere, yet the science was taking me was far afield from the masses. I thought if I was correct, the information could make a big difference to many people. So, my thoughts had to become actions, and I had to make some key decisions regarding proof.

To show biologic plausibility of my arguments, I knew I was going to have to show this link between leptin and pain could be useful clinically. I also realized that Shoemaker and conventional medicine did not realize the enormous potential of these links. So I had to lay it out on the line publicly, and I knew the Paleo elitists would scream bloody murder when I challenged their dogma. Their response was what I was hoping for.

HOW A THOUGHT BECOMES AN ACTION

Sometimes to transform we have to erase all we believe and begin anew.

I reflected on my knee injury and realized why my knee pain went away post-operatively as I lost weight and my HS-CRP fell. It increased my alpha-MSH to block the peripheral and central pathways of pain in my own nervous system. Not only is leptin yoked to light cycles, but it also is yoked to seasonal geothermal cycles via inflammatory cytokines. It was my eureka moment. I remember the day I realized it like it was yesterday. I now felt I could interpret many unexplainable things because of this insight.

I realized that I could have further increased my pain relief and fat loss by living in a cold environment at the same time. Our bodies make and modulate inflammatory cytokines different ways in different environments. I knew the wiring for cold adaptation was built into our DNA because of our ancestral history. I even gained some insight on why anorexia and bulimia might occur, based on these links with the leptin receptor.

THE REALIZATION OF A MAJOR PROBLEM

At this point, I knew I had to try and prove this on a patient with chronic pain of Neolithic disease, such as degenerative disc disease and disc herniation, to see if it could block the pain. There was one large problem.

How could I do this on a human without going through the Institutional Review Board (IRB) for permission? None of this science was proven or laid out in any textbook. It was a giant thought experiment supported by a ton of disparate facts. I was just connecting the dots and writing it all down in my Quilt document. I knew it was also written down in our DNA, but that is not the currency a clinician needs to experiment on humans! Even if I did manage to try this on a patient, my colleagues would have thought I was on the fringe because none of them knew how these bits of information fit into our biology. So I went back to the plastic surgery literature and the research on Zeltiq. By this time, my brother-in-law was interested in what I had learned and decided to see how the Zeltiq procedure worked on his abdomen. I was very interested in his results, and called him often during this time. He told me it shrank a bit of fat over six weeks, but that it had made him numb for close to six weeks after the treatments. I was more interested in that finding. Although he was disappointed, I was excited by this news, but never shared why. I knew I had to find a patient to test this hypothesis, so I got an idea to run several thought and lab experiments in early 2010 using my quantified self-testing platform.

I knew I could not test this hypothesis on a patient, but I could test it on myself without anyone's permission. I remembered in medical school learning about Barry Marshall and his theory of what caused gastric ulcers. At the time, medicine's standard of treatment for ulcers was to section the vagus nerve by the stomach to decrease acid production and decrease ulcer formation. I cannot tell you how many patients I saw this operation performed on, and looking back, it was pure nuts. It is an operation born of pure reductive thought with no insight into how it might inflict serious collateral damage. This is how I feel today about bariatric surgery, too.

Marshall was convinced through his own research that a bacteria called H. pylori caused gastric ulcers. Marshall traced not just ulcers, but also stomach cancer to this gut infection. The cure, he realized, was readily available: antibiotics (or the use of bismuth). But mainstream gastroenterologists and general surgeons dismissed his theories, holding on to the idea that stress caused ulcers. There was also a good business around the vagotomy operations for ulcers. Because no one believed him, Marshall had to find a novel way to prove his theory. Since he was unable to make his case with lab mice (because H. pylori affects only primates) and because he was prohibited from experimenting on people, Marshall finally ran an experiment on the only patient he could ethically recruit: himself. He swallowed the bacteria, became quite ill with gastritis, and eradicated the bacteria with antibiotics, thus proving his theory. I remembered this and thought, how could I prove acute leptin resistance increases surgical and chronic pain? The experiment would confirm cold could control appetite and narcotic use. I also thought it may have implications for longevity research, and help victims of bariatric surgery whose weight loss had plateaued once again lose weight, regardless of what was done to the vagus nerve in surgery. I felt a large amount of people could be helped with health problems paramount in our world today.

THE THOUGHT EXPERIMENT THEORY EXPLAINED

I was convinced that cold temperatures could restore leptin sensitivity quickly and reverse acute surgical pain by raising alpha-MSH and lowering IL-6. I decided to use Marshall's idea and use myself as the test subject.

I knew that leptin was yoked to light cycles and energy production, but I also believed it was linked to temperature. I felt that the link to temperature grew stronger as environmental light dropped in fall and winter. I thought cold could protect us from pain by making us extremely leptin sensitive. The side effects of this would be natural weight loss, decreased thirst, and no appetite. I wanted to tap the Epi-paleo Rx for pain control in our owner's manual. I believed evolution had to a plan for life to live on reduced pain, and that we could harness this power to help folks today. The implications of this theory could help millions of people with chronic pain, diabetic neuropathy, and acute or chronic surgically induced pain.

Since I happen to be in a specialty of medicine that inflicts surgical pain often, I became quite intrigued with this idea for the last several years. Could we use cold to make calorie restriction a viable option for the masses and extend our lifespan? I would have never been led down this pathway were it not for curing my own obesity. In the case of diabetic neuropathy, there is no good therapy available at all. The same is true for patients with chronic pain due to damaged nervous systems. Ever since I met those two women online, I thought about the links of fat atrophy and cold insensibility that were known but rarely correlated to other clinical conditions that could help people.

To prove my theory, I developed a plan in May 2011 to reverse engineer my own Leptin Rx and make myself acutely leptin resistant in about four to six weeks. I thought this would make me very susceptible to pain after an acute surgical situation. I thought it would be easy to do based on Linda Frassetto's paper on kidney patients at UCSF, mentioned earlier in the book. I thought if kidney failure patients could show positive responses after two weeks on a Paleo diet, I could cause leptin resistance pretty quickly by eating wheat and PUFAs. I worked it out in my head and visited a plastic surgeon in October 2011 for a consult. I only qualified for an elective procedure since I was pretty healthy, so I was limited to removal of my wisdom teeth or plastic surgery. I already had my wisdom teeth taken out in dental school, so decided to pick a plastic surgery procedure that would hurt pretty badly to disprove my hypothesis.

Anyone who knows me well knows I do not advocate plastic surgery because any surgery is potentially dangerous. I knew I could not tell my wife what I was up to either. I did give a few friends bits and pieces of information a few days before surgery, but not the whole plan. I told Bulletproof Executive Dave Asprey a couple of parts of this hack but not the surgery part. I also told Mark Sisson and Kevin Cottrell that I needed surgery to repair a torn rectus muscle (not true), but none of the details I am describing here now. If this worked, I wanted to save the story for this book, or bury it as a bad idea! I never told anyone in my family what I planned to do until December 15, 2011.

I dropped it on my wife and told her I wanted some work done on my chest, back, and abdomen. I never told her how extensive I was going to go with it because I did not want to scare her. Moreover, I knew I did not actually need work and was going to have to put on some fat to have removed to test the hypothesis. Basically, I was going to have unnecessary surgery to cause a lot of pain. Since I learned about the Zeltiq procedure in detail and how it worked, I went to visit a plastic surgeon friend I used to work with. I had not seen him in quite some time and he was shocked at how much weight I lost. I told him I wanted to be better sculpted, and I made sure he knew the surgery had to be extensive. I told him this because plastic surgeons are results-oriented, so I knew this meant he would be aggressive. I did this because it would hurt a lot more than a standard procedure. I did not tell him why I was doing the surgery because then he would never operate. This surgery was going to be my proof that extreme cold temperature alone could acutely reverse leptin resistance to control pain, without the use of narcotic drugs. I felt if I could show it worked on me, it might some day be used safely in surgery and other applications.

He looked me over and said I did not need any surgery, but that if I really wanted it, he would do it. For the next six weeks prior to the operation on January 9, 2012, I ate a diet that I knew would cause acute leptin resistance, increased post-op pain, and added fat. I put on about 17 pounds rather easily. My diet was loaded with whole grains, PUFAs, "safe starches," and dairy products. I specifically choose January 9 because 13 years earlier on that day I witnessed the most amazing thing. The Tennessee Titans beat the Buffalo Bills with 16 seconds left in a play. It was known as the Music City Miracle. I was hoping that some magic might repeat itself that day for me, too.

I went back and re-read the Zeltiq literature and the synthetic leptin data to make sure I was not missing any key points. I ate until my fasting blood glucose was over 88 consistently. This meant I was leptin resistant and had lost control of PEPCK, the enzyme gatekeeper for gluconeogensis. I ate like this for another two weeks for added proof. I also knew leptin resistance increased my chances of post-op acute pain. My plan was not to take any pain-relieving or sedative drugs except anesthesia to put me under for five hours. I refused all pre-op medications and made the nurses turn off the lights in pre-op holding area while I waited to be cut on at 9 a.m. I could see a lot of confused faces in the surgery center personnel because they knew how anti-plastic surgery I was. These were people I had worked with a long time and who knew how I felt about leptin and weight loss. I even mentioned to one of the nurses that I was performing a big experiment on myself and she looked perplexed, but did not question me further.

I woke up in the surgery center recovery area in some serious pain-a 10 of 10! First it was a dull ache, but as I came to it became intense and I quickly began to suffer. This I precisely what I expected after making myself leptin resistant during the prior six weeks, increasing my IL-6 and HS-CRP levels. I was not sure how the subcutaneous removal of fat would affect my hypothalamic response. It was pretty dramatic. I had severe thirst and had to urinate threes time in an hour. I also had an intense craving to eat something sweet about an hour into recovery. These were symptoms a diabetic might have. After my knee scope I had no thirst, was able to function easily, and never needed narcotics for pain. I also recalled I could not urinate post-op back then, too.

I continued to refuse all pain medicine and my wife was wondering why, because she saw I was in severe pain. It was then I told her what I had done. She was not too happy with me but she gathered me up and took me home. The day before I loaded the freezer with 120 pounds of ice. As soon as I got home at 3 p.m. I struggled into bed and immediately put 60 pounds of ice on the surgical areas.

Within five minutes I was completely numb and pain free! I went from a 10 out of 10 to a one out of 10. I was able to walk around, although with much difficulty. Within 20 minutes something else occurred that I did not expect. I started to become numb in areas of my skin that had no surgical scars or ice on them. My thirst went away, along with my hunger and appetite. I also became very sleepy after the ice was added to my body and slept soundly until 7:42 p.m. that night, when Richard Nikoley, of Free the Animal fame, returned a call.

I think I crashed hard because the lowering of IL-6 with cold can induce sleep, since insomnia is associated with high IL-6 levels. This is why cold helps induce hibernation, I think, in bears. The ice significantly lowered my IL-6, making me quite sleepy. Rich sensed something was wrong because I could barely speak due to the cold, and he asked me if I was OK. I told him that I was doing the biggest N=1 of my entire life (an N=1 is a trial in which a single patient is the entire trial). He told me he had done something similar once, but with a disc herniation in his neck. He told me that Kurt Harris turned him on to John Sarno's work and book and asked me if I was familiar with it. I told him I was and believed it could work, but by then I could not talk much because of the cold. I was shivering and found deep breathing tough, which made talking hard. I jotted down these thoughts on my laptop as soon as he hung up and fell back to sleep. Breathing was a bit rough when I was talking to Rich, but I was otherwise quite comfortable. I believe the ice brought my skin temperature down to 50-55 degrees at that time. It dropped even lower as I slept. I had a temperature gauge on my chest to make sure it was cold enough, and I was buck naked to give the ice full effect. I never took any pain medicine during this hack. The only thing I did was support my hormonal response for wound healing, which I knew would be down regulated by the elevated cortisol levels from a painful surgery. I took 25,000 IU of vitamin D3, 200 mg of pregenelone, 200 mg of Prometrium (progesterone), and 500 mg of DHEA.

I had planned to stay packed in the ice bath for 12 hours during the night and then acutely reverse the process by removing the ice at 3 a.m. and going without ice or medication for 12 hours. I felt this would induce my leptin resistance, increase IL-6, and induce an acute pregnenolone steal, which would increase pain, and that cold therapy would reverse the pain and leptin resistance if the ice treatment truly was effective post-operatively. I believed the ice would significantly raise my alpha-MSH while simultaneously lowering my leptin and IL-6 levels to control my pain without the use of exogenous narcotics.

THE RESULTS OF MY HACK: DID ACTIVATING FACTOR X WORK FOR ME?

As soon as the ice hit me after coming home from the hospital, I believe my IL-6 levels dropped, as my cravings for water and sweets quickly vanished. This replicated what astronauts and Sherpas reported when exposed to extreme cold. My deep thirst went away in 15 minutes. I believe this was due to modulation of antidiuretic hormone (ADH) secretion from the acute cytokine reduction. I also thought that this would help my blood loss because low ADH levels are associated with bleeding. So if my ADH levels increased I would experience no excess bleeding and would not need compression dressings. I found this to be exactly what happened.

The most amazing finding was that my pain went away totally in a few minutes and I was completely numb in areas where no surgery was performed within 15 minutes. I noticed the upper parts of my legs covering L1-L3 dermatomes became insensate (numb). I think this was because the drop of IL-6 and the surge of alpha-MSH shut down my lumbosacral plexus. I was very surprised areas that had no ice on them became numb. Honestly, I did not anticipate this benefit. During my recovery the next two weeks, I opened up my neurosurgery textbooks and figured out this actually made sense. I began to think about how the pain tracts are hardwired in the spinal cord and how this effect could be useful in the treatment of chronic pain from all causes. The numbers of patients suffering from chronic pain are staggering just in the United States alone. Worldwide, the numbers are mind-boggling.

I began to shiver pretty violently but then it stopped after about 10 minutes. I think the shivering was due to activation of my UCP 1, 2 and 3, because the monitor showed my surface body temp sunk quickly to 55 degrees. We know that levels of UCP1 mRNA are increased three- to fourfold after just four hours of exposure. I think because I had been very cold-adapted pre-operatively, it happened even quicker. At this point I became very sleepy and fell asleep.

I had set my clock for 3 a.m. for the second part of the test and instructed my wife to replenish my ice when it melted. I was not looking forward to part two of this test-I had to make sure leptin and temperature caused these effects, not some other factor. I woke up at 3 a.m. quite comfortable and removed all the ice. I stayed comfortable for about 45 minutes, but then the dull pain returned, followed by very sharp pain around 4 a.m. The hours between 4 a.m. and 6 a.m. were the worst two hours of my life. It was horrible. My wife woke up to find me in tears and asked if I want pain medication, but I declined. I asked for ice immediately. I told her there was no way I could make it nine more hours without the ice. I was a giant "wussy" for sure. She packed me with 40 more pounds of ice and I had complete pain relief for the next six hours. I learned a lot in this N=1 experiment.

THE IMPLICATIONS OF THIS SUCCESS

I think my case made it clear that patients with acute or chronic leptin resistance are far more susceptible to pain. As a neurosurgeon, this has huge implications for my practice, and even bigger implications for medicine and anesthesia. I have noticed in the many surgical cases I have done over the last 10 years that diabetics and people with fibromyalgia require a lot more narcotics for surgery. Instead of withholding medication, I needed to use cold temperature modulation to quickly extend pain relief. The more unresolved pain they had, the worse their pregnenolone steal would be and the longer recovery would take. I have newfound insight as to why they recover so much more slowly than those who do not have co-morbid leptin issues and I know I can introduce ideas to help them recover quicker. I also know the more leptin resistant someone is pre-op the more difficult it is for them to overcome any surgery, painful or not. Moreover, as surgeons, we need to be mindful of this when we operate on people who are obese, anorexic, or on medication for chronic pain.

I was truly amazed at how well the ice worked in this surgical application. Most surgeons will find it hard to believe because many of us have used ice before, but not to this degree. We need to design ways to use it more effectively pre-operatively. Most of us do not live in the tundra, but for 10 days post-op I created a cold, dark Neolithic "Arctic Zone" in my house and around my body. Moreover, its onset of action was much faster than narcotics. I think someone in deep pain from a stroke, an amputation, any damage of the spinal cord, or a partial nerve injury would have little problem tolerating the coldness if it meant pain relief, even without doing the practice runs with ice packing I did prior to this experiment. For me, I would have jumped in the Arctic Ocean for pain relief during those two hours after surgery when I removed the ice from my torso. I wondered if this is why some people join Polar Bear Clubs, not understanding why it makes them feel better. The key is delivering enough coldness over a period of time to make it worthwhile for both the surgical period and for patients with chronic pain. I also believe this will help surgical patients recover quicker because it allows normal hormonal responses to return faster, as the cold therapy controls all the major inflammatory cytokines that underpin poor surgical recoveries. I have never had such fast relief from any pain medication in my life. I think the implications of this bio-hack are huge and may form the Epi-paleo Rx for all chronic pain patients.

Perhaps we could develop custom-fitted cooling blankets with built-in temperature sensors to help those with diabetic neuropathy or myelopathy. It may allow people with pain from thalamic strokes to be treated without brain surgery. People with phantom limb pain may be able to alleviate pain using temperature modulation at home without much medical intervention. Other potential treatment populations include people with anesthesia dolorous, or trigeminal neuralgia. This is a nerve disorder that causes such severe pain it's called "suicide disease" because so many of its victims commit suicide. What about the people for whom a gastric bypass failed? I might have just stumbled upon a new tool for their success, too. We might be able to decrease narcotic dependency in all pain clinics. My two weeks of recovery were bittersweet! I was pumped that my thought experiment was a smashing success, but when I looked at my badly bruised torso in the mirror or my wife's face, I was blindsided by emotion.

I think the most exciting question is how this might help longevity. If coldness can immediately raise alpha-MSH and decrease leptin and inflammatory cytokines, we maybe able to create the perfect scenario for longevity, which is encouraged by by low inflammation and increased telomere lengths. We know Sherpas eat a lot less food and have naturally lower metabolisms because they have lived in cold areas for the last 25,000 years. Using cold temperatures, we can not only lower inflammation, but also naturally induce calorie restriction because of cold's modulating effects on leptin. Sherpas and astronauts have already shown us this phenomena in NASA tests. One of the major problems in longevity research is that calorie restriction is hard to implement because it stimulates appetite and hunger. I found in my hack that cold destroys appetite while naturally selecting for a calorie-restricted Paleolithic diet. If I were a longevity researcher, I would be moving my primates and humans as far north or south as possible or temperature controlling their environment to conduct research. I also think cold will give us results faster than we expect.

A PROPOSED MECHANISM OF THE HCG DIET NOW EXPLAINED? THE HOLY TRINITY

The HCG diet and calorie restriction are two ways to activate parts of this ancient survival pathway. The only part that is missing is the cold environment. I realized this on post op-day three. It made perfect sense why both worked, but only partially. HCG destroys hunger on 500 calories but cannot sustain long-term weight loss, while calorie restriction works great if you can stand being hungry the rest of your life. If you just change one thing-the temperature of the environment-everything works perfectly. The Holy Trinity is a massive blog that lays out how calorie-restricted diets, HCG, and cold therapy form the key elements of the ancient mammalian for survival. You can find that here http://jackkruse.com/the-holy-trinity-ct-4/

HCG modulates our thyroid function to decrease our body temperature while simultaneously increasing our endogenous opioid production to increase fat burning. It might do this while we are burning calories as free heat, uncoupled from our mitochondria, via UCP1 and UCP3. If these calories are uncoupled from the mitochondria, it likely will lengthen our telomere lengths. This is now an experiment that anyone can do to see if it works. It would not take long and it would be easy to measure telomere lengths on leukocytes.

PRIMAL PEOPLE CAN EXPERIMENT AND PROVE IT FOR THEMSELVES AT HOME NOW

I think this has huge implications because temperature-regulated blankets to produce a cold environment for the body can be used at home for many different patients, requiring no special hospital equipment. It also appears the anesthetic effects are generalized over the body and not just the areas covered by cold therapy, so it will help cover wider areas of the painful regions. This also would not require an NIH grant or FDA approval. This is something the general public could do to see if it helps modulate their pain without drugs. Patients with chronic pain would be the ideal testers. I found the pain control became more effective the more time I used it, and the pain relief lasted longer without any ice. I am sure there is a mathematical reason, but I am not smart enough to figure that out right now. I do, however, believe I can explain it. I believe this occurred because the brain began immediately rewiring to adapt to cold stimuli. I think this is an evolutionary adaptation that makes sense when we consider the rapid onset of ice ages humans have faced over the last 2.5 million years.

Based on my reading, scientists believe there have been at least five major ice ages in the earth's past. My bet is there were more because data from one ice age is lost as the next one occurs. I base this on something I learned in a NOVA program in 2005 called, The Big Chill. Here is an excerpt from that amazing documentary: "Ever since the Pre-Cambrian explosion (670 million years ago), ice ages have occurred at widely spaced intervals of geologic time-approximately 200 million years-lasting for millions, or even tens of millions of years. For the Cenozoic period, which began about 70 million years ago and continues today, evidence derived from marine sediments provides a detailed, and fairly continuous, record for climate change. This record indicates decreasing deep-water temperature, along with the build-up of continental ice sheets. Much of this deep-water cooling occurred in three major steps about 36, 15 and 3 million years ago-the most recent of which continues today." Moreover, today 90 percent of the living biome still lives in a cold environment on our planet! Maybe we are just unaware of how different living is for us today compared to our ancestors?

The program went on to say, "During the present ice age, glaciers have advanced and retreated over 20 times, often blanketing North America with ice. Our climate today is actually a warm interval between these many periods of glaciation. The most recent period of glaciation, which many people think of as the 'Ice Age,' was at its height approximately 20,000 years ago."

Modern geologic science reconstructs ice age formations by relying on data that was often displaced or destroyed by subsequent ice ages. More definitive scientific proof is, I believe, hardwired into our leptin receptor and how we account for food as a species. I bet any animal we test this hypothesis on will have the same results because our cells, and all animal cells today, came from ancestors who navigated these conditions successfully. This may be a place where evolutionary biology supports modern geologic theory.

Please consider this. What if we're dead wrong and our biochemistry is best adapted for cold environments yet we live in a warm world? What if a cold environment is our primordial condition? What if Mother Nature's plans differ from the modern life we have created? Scientists believe we are in an ice age today and at the end of a warming cycle that began 11,000 years ago. We know of 11 warming periods that have occurred since we evolved. What if I told you that your proteins and enzymes react completely opposite in a cold environment? This is detailed in the cold thermogenesis series on my website.

Maybe modern life is the ultimate biologic mismatch to the blueprint evolution used to help us survive the K-T event. Ninety percent of life on Earth today still lives in those cold environments deep in our oceans and seas, on the tundra, and in the polar regions. Evolutionary biologists will tell you that the living biome 67 million years later still is following that plan! It appears the animals from back then have adapted to a far different environment while the evolution of their species has greatly sped up. This is the perfect Rx for Neolithic disease. Take a look at modern humans. Our species in the Western world is in decline. We epitomize mediocrity. Our health falls apart in midlife because of these mismatches. And my prediction is even more dire. As evolution speeds forward so will our epigenetics. This is why we see diabetic children today. Modern life is not safe for us. In fact, the convenience of modern life may bankrupt us before it extinguishes us. Our health care system is designed to keep us sick instead of getting us well, and our brain's innovations further speed evolution to create more mismatches that might kill us! We go to the doctor today to get a pill for every ill while we get a wallet biopsy. There appear to be no answers for many of Neolithic diseases by the complex that is supposed to care for us. How crazy is this? Americans need to help themselves to avoid my profession as much as they can, otherwise they subjugate themselves to a brutal system that will enslave them in illness.

Here is another possibility we may not be aware of. Does this mean the African savanna is not what shaped human evolution as we believe today? Epigenetic science tells us what happened in previous generations is more important that we know. This implies the sicker we get the weaker the species becomes. We are basically extinguishing ourselves! For optimal function, evidence points to a nutrient dense, ketogenic Paleolithic diet rich in fish, protein, and fats; cold environments for good cell membrane signaling; and perfect ratios of EFAs in our cell membranes. Modern biochemistry in textbooks today is based on warm-adapted pathways and it is not completely correct in my opinion. If one considers the frostbite data done at Harvard and if one spoke to the Zeltiq engineers at Mass General, you would find the hominid biochemistry of fat loss in cold environments makes fat accumulation impossible in cold-adapted, land-based mammals. The main reason is because of how epigenetics is handled at the cellular membrane. Cold-adapted, water-based mammals need a much lower omega 6 to 3 ratio of fatty acids to function. More double bonds in omega 3s allow for better membrane fluidity and cell membrane signaling the colder it gets. Cold water conducts heat away from the body 24 times faster than cold air, so cold-adapted water mammals have different epigenetic signaling for fat mass than cold-adapted land mammals.

Land-based mammals need an omega 6 to 3 ratio at 4/1. If the ratio is off, the biology of the adipocytes change. I think Johns Hopkins researcher Patricia Kane's 35 years of work on the lipid layers covering cells backs this up. Animals (including humans) cannot produce the polyunsaturated lipids, which have more than one double bond. Omega 6 EFAs, or linoleic acid (LA), and omega 3 EFAs, or alpha linoleic acid (ALA), are produced by land and ocean plants. All of our cells require these two EFAs and they must be included in sufficient quantities in the diet. Although the science of fats and oils is still unclear in regards to cell membrane function, we know their importance is paramount to life in different environments on our planet. There is probably no dietary requirement more critical than the ingestion of the correct ratio of EFAs, which research has shown in cold adapted mammals to be 4 parts omega 6 to one part omega 3. The polar seas provide mammals with massive amounts of krill to get to a 1/1 ratio, necessary for a life lived almost in total winter at the poles or in the deep sea. Land-based plants and protein sources provide for a proper 4/1 ratio for cold-adapted land mammals. This is seen in polar bears, Bactrian camels, and humans! Unfortunately, it no longer applies to the Inuit of the polar regions.

Since the 1950s, the Inuit are no longer cold-adapted. Transportation has brought them a modern, warm diet. We can read the accounts of what the Inuit looked like from Schweitzer, Price, or Vilhjalmur Stefansson (1879-1962), who spent 11 years living among the Inuit. He was adopted into an Inuit family, lived in a tent, and ate fish and seal meat, often raw or fermented. He concluded that he had never been in better health in his life. He also writes about the excellent health, including dental health, and the absence of headaches experienced on exclusive animal-foods diet. You can find his account of what a human life is like being cold adapted here: http://www.drbass.com/stefansson2.html.

Modern scientists understand warm-adapted mammalian biochemistry, but remain blind to the fact that land-based mammals have both a warm and cold pathway tied to circadian biology. There are many biochemical experts today, but all of them have been educated by books written after 1950, and all of these books are based on warm-adapted humans.

I do not believe that scientists know or believe that humans have a thermoplastic biochemistry like other mammals. This is what allows mammals to enter the cold pathways when the climate changes. If you do not know this and apply the warm biochemistry principles to experiments on mammals, you might end up with the belief that cold causes subcutaneous fat deposition. This is precisely why modern scientists believe ketosis is not a good long-term strategy. Most very low-carb (VLC) dieters have bad body composition eating this way because they are warm adapted. It happens because the VLC diet requires a cold-adapted environment to work optimally. If one is warm-adapted and eats VLC, you become "skinny fat," developing subcutaneous fat and not muscle.

Moreover, cold-adapted land mammals have different epigenetic controls over adipocytes than water-based mammals. Patricia Kane's research elucidates evolutionary reasons why cold-adapted cell membrane biology is quite different. This is why whales and walrus have to eat huge amounts of krill and fish each day to tolerate the cold deep oceans. This affects their fat cells differently than PUFAs do. It is also why I warn my blog readers not to go hog wild with omega three supplements, and why I disagree with many fish oil calculators in the Paleo 1.0 books.

Cold-adapted water mammals have different mechanisms that allow for fat protection. Evolution went from sea to land, and we come from those water-based ancestors. The primates we came from use biochemistry that was naturally selected for by the environments they faced. This means the leptin receptor and its pathways became adapted to warm environments over time. We can live warm adapted today, but not optimally because our metabolism is still suited best to fat burning in cold environments. When I see people comparing my theory to cold-adapted water mammals they are missing the evolutionary adaptations that life made when it came out of the water and onto land. This is why cold-adapted land mammals are the best comparison.

It appears evolution says the path to survival is the epigenetic program it created after the K-T event, which got us here today. The K-T event was the major factor that sped up mammalian epigenetics to offset a slower reproductive rate found in our cold polar regions. It is Factor X. This was controlled by the power laws of mathematics and guaranteed our species its best chance for survival.

In fact, in 67 million years, the leptin-melanocortin ancient pathway brought us from small hibernating mammals to what we are today. The K-T event was the fuel that sped up the evolutionary epigenetic process compared to other epochs. This is another consequence of this genetic program. Evolutionary biologists will tell you biologic programs get extinguished pretty rapidly if they are not useful. The fact that cold thermogenesis is still within our brains and is rapidly inducible in anyone who attempts it is a testament to its importance to all mammalian life. I think it extends all the way back to life's genesis, but was sculpted by 4.5 billion years of cold adaptations. Moreover, we need to be mindful of how it might affect us today, in a world opposite to what our genome is best adapted to for survival. The implications of this new reality are nothing short of startling for modern chronic diseases.

Think of it this way: when you think of a sport car's introduction to the public, everyone knows it was made for power and speed. After some years, an oil crisis suddenly turns everyone's attention to cars that are more energy efficient. The public makes adjustments to survive market pressures. When the market stabilizes, things revert to the norm and car engineers adjust design to meet market demand. What is the moral of the story? In the beginning a Porsche was a Porsche, and after the oil crisis it is still a Porsche, holding true to its origins. Although it evolves, it still relies on its original blueprint of power and speed. Humans are no different than those eutherian mammals were 67 million years ago. Even our biochemistry acts that way when forced. We do not need to use the survival blueprint today because we do not face what they faced. But the capability is there. And it is a program that evolution sculpted to see that we SURVIVE IT. You reading this book is the best proof of this.

The leptin-melanocortin ancient pathway is nothing short of amazing for all mammals. It turns mammals into super athletes to tackle survival when food is scarce and the world is frozen. We are all products of that experiment, and the Optimal Rx calls for you to live in congruency with that blueprint today.

Because of the rapidity to which my nervous system responded to the cold stimuli after surgery, my brain began rewiring immediately to account for this because the biologic program is already built into us. This was climate change inducing a long-lost program. As a neurosurgeon, this rapidity of adaptation flies in the face of what I was taught. It is nothing short of amazing.

What I learned in my recovery is that we can quickly train the brain out of chronic pain if we just favorably alter its environment. It is brain surgery without a scalpel, using nothing but cold. Eventually, it also did not take as much cold as it did initially for the same effect. As soon as I perceived the temperature change it seemed to really stop the pain effectively and quickly. It was as if my brain rewired itself to the cold stimuli to stop the pain as fast as it could to help me adapt. This made biologic sense to me as I wondered how life adapted to the ice ages in years past.

I paid attention to my skin color to see if it got darker due to upregulation of alpha-MSH, but I am fair-skinned and never tan, so I may not be a good person to test this. The elevated ACTH expanded my well-being, which helped me heal quite fast. I did not do a blood test because it was not practical, and I did not want to do much traveling considering how beat up I was. I did not use one pain pill during the entire recovery process, but I went through a lot of ice!

I do think the cold stimulus rapidly decreased the inflammatory cytokine response. I think life in general is explained through our cytokine response and hormonal tests. The most obvious thing my family noticed was how my appetite and hunger went away when I was packed in ice but it returned as soon as I removed it. I think adding ice baths to the Leptin Rx reset is something that will benefit all people, and is ideal for those who have sustained bariatric damage to their vagus nerve. They need cold to fully reverse their obesity. Diabetics and those on HCG would also expect to see increased results with cold. In fact, this explains why evolution allows for diabetes to occur.

Mammals became diabetic by eating summer fruits. Insulin resistance made them sluggish, signaling them to find a den underground and hibernate. As they hibernated through the winter, their fat loss allowed them to remain insensate to the cold, kept their immune systems strong, and drove down Il-6 levels. Low IL-6 selected for high DHEA, which is correlated with great sleep. Everything is a perfect biologic fit and explains how mammals survive winter normally. I think using temperature to quickly lose weight and reset the hypothalamus is not only possible, but very likely the best way to reverse metabolic syndrome.

I now add cold to the Leptin Rx reset to induce this ancient pathway faster to restore health. This will take some training for the public. It took me six months to be able to tolerate 12 hours of this kind of cold. I did find I progressively became thirstier during the first week after surgery. I am not sure if this was dehydration from the anesthesia and the surgical recovery or an effect of the chronic cooling. My sleep also improved with the application of ice throughout the first week, which I expected thanks to declining IL-6 levels. I went back to my normal eating pattern post-op, but found restricting calories easier with the chronic use of cooling for pain control. At this writing, it has been three months since that biohack and I am still not back to normal. I have been using cold thermogenesis to lose the excess weight successfully but I am not back to feeling as I did last fall.

I plan to use this technique for my chronic pain patients, but I am also intrigued by its applications for longevity and weight loss. It appears this is a way to lower inflammation in the mTOR and IGF-1 pathways simultaneously no matter what we eat. I think the greatest effect will be combining it with a Paleolithic diet.

Modern health care is broken because it is divorced from the evolutionary theory that is foundational to its science. The same is not true for physics, chemistry, or geology. It is time we use evolution to guide our treatments, not the biased beliefs built into randomized control trials of the last 50 years. Look at what those trials have brought us today-mediocrity as a species. Evolution brought us from our primate ancestors to the most amazing creation of all life forms. Our own brains, however, have allowed for our slow destruction as we move away from Mother Nature's blueprint.

WHAT THE OPTIMAL RX CAN DO FOR US ALL RIGHT NOW

I now look at every disease using this Epi-paleo Rx as my new North Star. My next book will be a handbook for patients and physicians to use to guide them back to their own North Star using the tools I have shared with you here. I left many steps out. If you are told every last detail your learning would be suboptimal. If you do not believe me, read Malcom Gladewell's book, Blink. I designed my Quilt document on my website to do the same thing to your brain. Thirty levees are listed, but none are put together for you to see how all the information is connected. With every blog I post, the picture gets a bit clearer for the reader. As I add blogs, you come to your own awareness of what optimal really is based upon our biology. In that way you find the answer yourself and can then transform your thinking and your life. Total transformation requires you to become aware of something you were not aware of before. This is how the human brain learns best. Regular change does not metamorphosize our species, which is why humans rarely adapt when they know something is bad for them. Instead, they adapt when they become aware of something to which they were previously blind.

My plan is to rewire your thinking for a new understanding of how to change yourself and become the change you seek in medicine. We have been mediocre too long. We can teach each other the changes we seek in health care. These thoughts are my contribution to the people I let down during the last 20 years. All one has to do is apply the principles found in this book to find the answers you seek.

The simple fact is we spent hundreds of thousands of years adapting to a relatively narrow range of parameters in the ancestral environment, then to a few thousand years of Neolithic farming villages, and then to the last century or so of having completely redesigned our environment. This completely redesigned technological environment selects for pathological gene expression. This includes the food we eat, the technology we use, and others aspects of modern life. We must remain aware of how these things can hurt our genes, even though they are amazing creations of our brain and make life easier. However, evolution is not based upon making life easier. It is based upon natural selection for survival of the fittest. Recognition of this alone is the first step to optimal health. To return to optimal, we need to invoke what our evolution wired into us 67 million years ago. When you are cold-adapted in fall and winter, and eat a Paleolithic ketogenic diet that favors leptin sensitivity and low inflammation, you can avoid most modern disease. The diet provides the optimal four to one omega 6/3 ratio required for optimal cell membrane signaling in cold-adapted land mammals. In spring and summer, we can eat via a warm-adapted pathway, to which we also have adapted. The leptin receptor has undergone 67 million years of evolution to allow us to live this way in the correct times of year. If you live in this fashion, you will not succumb to the Neolithic diseases the masses now think are normal human aging. I reject that. My primal sense won't allow for it any longer.

I hope these Rxs help you and save you from any Neolithic hurdle you face from this day forward.

The next step in my evolution is completion of my own journey. I realized during the last two months of my recovery that practiced thinking is the hardest part of my learning, and that training my mind is the essence of my transformation.

As I like to say on the Internet, "I ain't close to done yet." I hope this book becomes your proof that one thought might just change your DNA.

REFERENCES

1. http://discovermagazine.com/2010mar/07-dr-drank-broth-gave-ulcer-solved-medical-mystery
2. http://healthcare.utah.edu/publicaffairs/spotlight/SuperSherpa.html
3. Williams, D.M., Pollard, P. (2002). "Earth-like worlds on eccentric orbits: excursions beyond the habitable zone". Inter. J. Astrobio. 1: 21–9.
4. Kaufman, D.; Schneider, D.; McKay, N.; Ammann, C.; Bradley, R.; Briffa, K.; Miller, G.; Otto-Bliesner, B. et al. (2009). "Recent warming reverses long-term arctic cooling". Science 325 (5945): 1236–1239. Bibcode 2009Sci...325.1236K. doi:10.1126/science.1173983. PMID 19729653. edit
5. "Arctic Warming Overtakes 2,000 Years of Natural Cooling". UCAR. September 3, 2009. Retrieved 19 May 2011.

6. Bello, David (September 4, 2009). "Global Warming Reverses Long-Term Arctic Cooling". Scientific American. Retrieved 19 May 2011.

7. Richard A Muller, Gordon J. F. MacDonald (1997). "Glacial Cycles and Astronomical Forcing". Science 277 (5323): 215–8. Bibcode 1997Sci...277..215M. doi:10.1126/science.277.5323.215.

8. "Origin of the 100 kyr Glacial Cycle: eccentricity or orbital inclination?". Richard A Muller. Retrieved March 2, 2005.

9. Milankovitch, Milutin (1998) [1941]. Canon of Insolation and the Ice Age Problem. Belgrade: Zavod za Udzbenike i Nastavna Sredstva. ISBN 8617066199.

10. Roe G (2006). "In defense of Milankovitch". Geophysical Research Letters 33 (24): L24703. Bibcode 2006GeoRL..3324703R. doi:10.1029/2006GL027817. This shows that Milankovitch theory fits the data extremely well, over the past million years, provided that we consider derivatives.

11. Zachos J, Pagani M, Sloan L, Thomas E, Billups K (2001). "Trends, Rhythms, and Aberrations in Global Climate 65 Ma to Present". Science 292 (5517): 686–693. Bibcode 2001Sci...292..686Z. doi:10.1126/science.1059412. PMID 11326091.

12. Fortey, R (1999). Life: A Natural History of the First Four Billion Years of Life on Earth. Vintage. pp. 238–260. ISBN 978-0-375-70261-7.

13. Gradstein F, Ogg J, Smith A. A Geologic Time Scale 2004. ISBN 0521781426.

14. Alvarez et al. Extraterrestrial cause for the Cretaceous–Tertiary extinction Science 208, 6 June 1980. Retrieved: 26 May 2010.

15. Alvarez, LW, Alvarez, W, Asaro, F, and Michel, HV (1980). "Extraterrestrial cause for the Cretaceous–Tertiary extinction". Science 208 (4448): 1095–1108. Bibcode 1980Sci...208.1095A. doi:10.1126/science.208.4448.1095. PMID 17783054.

16. Padian K & Chiappe LM (1997). "Bird Origins". In Currie PJ & Padian K. Encyclopedia of Dinosaurs. San Diego: Academic Press. pp. 41–96.

17. Gauthier, J (1986). "Saurischian Monophyly and the origin of birds". In Padian K. The Origin of Birds and the Evolution of Flight. Mem. California Acad. Sci 8. pp. 1–55.

18. Hou L,Martin M, Zhou Z & Feduccia A, (1996) "Early Adaptive Radiation of Birds: Evidence from Fossils from Northeastern China" Science 274(5290): 1164-1167 Abstract

19. Huxley, T.H. (1876): Lectures on Evolution. New York Tribune. Extra. no 36. In Collected Essays IV: pp 46-138 original text w/ figures

20. Norell, M & Ellison M (2005) Unearthing the Dragon, The Great Feathered Dinosaur Discovery Pi Press, New York, ISBN 0-13-186266-9

21. J. Imbrie and K. P. Imbrie, Ice Ages: Solving the Mystery (Short Hills, NJ: Enslow Publishers) 1979.

22. Kuhle, M.(1988): The Pleistocene Glaciation of Tibet and the Onset of Ice Ages- An Autocycle Hypothesis. GeoJournal 17 (4, Tibet and High-Asia. Results of the Sino-German Joint Expeditions (I), 581-596.

23. Kuhle, M. (2004): The High Glacial (Last Ice Age and LGM) ice cover in High and Central Asia. Development in Quaternary Science 2c (Quaternary Glaciation - Extent and Chronology, Part III: South America, Asia, Africa, Australia, Antarctica, Eds: Ehlers, J.; Gibbard, P.L.), 175-199. (Elsevier B.V., Amsterdam)

24. Turpeinen, H.; Hampel, A.; Karow, T.; Maniatis, G. (2008). "Effect of ice sheet growth and melting on the slip evolution of thrust faults". Earth and Planetary Science

25. http://www.pbs.org/wgbh/nova/earth/cause-ice-age.html

26. Bottke, W.F.; Vokrouhlicky, D., Nesvorny, D. (September 2007). "An asteroid breakup 160 Myr ago as the probable source of the K/T impactor" (PDF). Nature 449 (7158): 23–25. Bibcode 2007Natur.449...48B. doi:10.1038/nature06070. PMID 17805288. Retrieved 2007-10-03.

27. Alvarez, W.; L.W. Alvarez, F. Asaro, and H.V. Michel (1979). "Anomalous iridium levels at the Cretaceous/Tertiary boundary at Gubbio, Italy: Negative results of tests for a supernova origin". In Christensen, W.K., and Birkelund, T.. Cretaceous/Tertiary Boundary Events Symposium. 2. University of Copenhagen. pp. 69.

Appendix A

THE EPI-PALEO RX DIET

The K-T event radically changed the world when the ascension of eutherian mammals ended the dominance of non-avian dinosaurs. It is unknown how long life had to subsist on a marine diet in the freezing cold, but one thing is crystal clear: we are here as proof of its success. What is not so clear is the path that leads from primitive mammals to modern humans. That is a story for another day, but the data of our origins is taking shape. Genomic studies show we came from transitional apes (transitional creatures between apes and humans) in the East African Rift zone, a place where three tectonic plates meet. The area has seen amazing geologic change over the last 10 million years, shifting from a hot tropical forest to a cool seacoast environment. I detail these dramatic climate changes in a post called Brain Gut 4 on my blog at www.jackkruse.com. This transition mimicked the abrupt changes of the K-T event, creating a cold environment that required adaptation to marine food for survival and spurred a change in species.

It appears the events surrounding the East African Rift zone created the ability to access the ancient survival pathway originally sculpted by the K-T event. I believe it was the immediate access to nutritionally rich marine food that allowed the simpler primate to evolve into a human who walked on two legs and had a more complex brain. It seems unbelievable until you understand the science of neural lipid biology, DHA, and iodine. When these brain-specific nutrients came together in the diet it created a perfect storm for the creation of the human brain. I laid this all out in a blog called Brain Gut 5 at my website as well. It is not easy reading, but the science is there with cites to many authors and researchers who have seen the connection between human brain evolution and the marine food chain. Our species was built around a marine diet and the amount of support for this assertion is growing. Understanding the unique attributes of the human brain helps reveal how these events likely unfolded.

IODINE

The thyroid hormones thyroxine (T4) and triiodothyronine (T3) are synthesized from iodine and play a crucial role in human evolution. T3 was critical not only for the evolution of the human brain but also for the ability to walk upright on two legs (bipedalism). Transitional apes already possessed hind limbs, however they lengthened under the influence of massive dietary iodine from marine foods. This is why bipedalism appears in the fossil record before the increase in brain size. The bone collectors still argue over this because they do not understand the implications of human brain evolution. They must stop looking at our evolution from bone data and begin to look at what truly separates us from transitional apes-our central nervous system. That can drive us to ask better questions about where we really came from.

The bone collectors found hominid fossils in places where fresh water and land would have met in the East African Rift and in South Africa. We also know the migration out of Africa took place largely on coastlines. Together these environments link early humans to seafood and vegetable diets rich in iodine, iron, vitamins A, vitamin D, and DHA. As humans move away from the ancestral diet that formed our brains we see major nutrient deficiencies, with vitamin D being the most obvious today. Iodine deficiency also affects a billion people today. Most people in the West eating a standard American diet are deficient in DHA. A diet low in DHA slows cognitive function and increases the risk of psychiatric illness.

Another interesting difference between apes and humans is seen in infancy. The chimp is born without much fat while a human baby is born with rolls of fat and an exceptional amount of brown fat. This extra fat allows fetal brain development to finish outside of the mother because the constraints of the human pelvis require birth before the baby's head grows too large. Also, the human brain is an energy hog and the extra fat at birth allows for the brain's energy requirements. A tremendous amount of subcutaneous fat helps the child form ketone bodies, an alternative fuel source for the brain. Ketones are important in infancy for another reason. The yet undeveloped infant brain lacks the protective myelin coating on the brain's main nerve fiber tracts. This is why an infant cannot walk or be self-sufficient. In fact, infants are born with primitive reflexes to compensate for this lack of myelination. Also, ketone bodies from infant fat help form brain-specific cholesterol and fatty acids vital to continued neurological development. Because ketones can't be stored they go straight to use for energy or construction, both of which are in high demand by the infant. A baby puts on most of its fat through the placenta in the last trimester of pregnancy.

One measure of an animal's relative intelligence is the encephalization quotient (EQ), or the ratio between brain mass and body mass. Other factors, such as the environment, also play a role in the EQ. For instance, in general carnivores have a higher EQ than herbivores because finding insect and animal prey for food requires more intelligence.

Lucy, one of humanity's early ancestors, walked upright, had ape and human features, and an EQ of 43 percent. Homo habilis came later, used stone tools, and had an EQ of 53 percent. Homo erectus, who looked similar to modern humans, existed around the same time as Homo habilis, but had an EQ of 63 percent and a larger body and brain (40 percent larger than Homo habilis). Next up was Homo heidelbergensis with an EQ of 75 percent, and then Homo neanderthalensis, with a larger brain and body but not a larger brain volume.

In fact, the largest hominid brain belongs not to us but to early modern humans, the Cro-Magnon, who shared the European continent for some time with Homo neanderthalensis. The Cro-Magnon brain weighed just over 3 pounds while the modern human brain weighs a few ounces less than that, and our bodies are smaller as well. Cro-Magnons, however, were smaller than Neanderthals.

Brain size is not necessarily a measure of cognitive potential. We know this because Neanderthals had larger brains than us by 10 percent but there is no evidence they had more cognitive ability. Instead, the primary area of evolution is the neocortex, which forms the top six layers of the human brain and allows for more expanded cognitive functions such as speech, comprehension, and calculations. Each layer has a specific function and morphology (shape).

Chimps retain the more Paleo functions of the visual cortex. Chimps have an amazing ability to track and remember visual cues compared to humans. Chimps can also see red better than we can-red pigments in leaves increase as the leaf gets older and is less nutritious to chimps, so they are able to avoid them. Humans have lost this ability. In essence, as the brain obtains special features it gives up others, becoming a Jack of all trades and master of none.

The ability to visually track and remember would be more important if you lived in a jungle with no stop signs or street signs. As humans developed the ability to speak it marginalized or extinguished the visual memory abilities we see in chimps. The cortex is expanded in humans to allow for verbal communication, which appears to have occurred in early Homo habilis.

Infant brains make up 11 percent of the child's weight while the adult brain makes up only 2-3 percent of body weight, giving the human infant a massive head-to-body ratio. The child's head passes through the birth canal only because the sutures of the skull are moldable and still open. This is a tightly controlled process in maternal fetal development and if the child's head is too big for the mother's pelvis it creates birthing problems. Neolithic disease such as gestational diabetes can create massive mismatches in both infant head size and pelvic size that can lead to the requirement of a C-section. This never happens in chimps.

Chimp babies are very lean compared to human infants and have brains that are 30 percent smaller. Chimp brains also do not grow much after birth whereas the human brain will triple in size during the first six years of life.

The most interesting thing about the human infant brain is its specific nutrient requirements. Infant brains are very sensitive to deficiencies in iodine and iron, sensitivities that remain until early adulthood. Early postnatal deficiencies in these nutrients can result in cretinism or developmental delay. Today, 20 percent of the earth's population has iodine or iron deficiencies and the further away from the oceans people live the more common these deficiencies are. If you have ever been to Nepal you might see goiters the size of basketballs.

The most startling gamble evolution made on the infant human brain is its massive energy requirements. The infant brain consumes an unbelievable 75 percent of the infant's energy. This ratio exceeds the adult human energy requirements by 300 percent. Children are also born helpless compared to chimps, further compounding the bet because this puts the mother at risk. This implies to me there had to be a massive pay off for these risks, and that the environment we evolved into had to provide massive resources for the child and mother. This points to an extremely nutrient-dense diet and a stable environment with limited insults to the brain during the 2 million years we evolved from Lucy.

The diet was rich in DHA, iron, and iodine, and the environment was cooler than normal. Cooler environments protect the brain from insults and can reduce its energy requirements by up to 25 percent. The brain takes up 20 percent of caloric energy while the heart, liver, and kidneys takes up 45 percent. To support brain energy, the gut would have had to shorten tremendously and develop the ability to dilate its vascular tree to support blood flow during eating and digestion. These are precisely the morphologic and physiologic adaptations we see in the human gut.

WHERE EVOLUTIONARY FORM MEETS EVOLUTIONARY FUNCTION?

Because the brain has no energy stores it has two ways to obtain fuel. One is glucose, which is not as efficient as ketones. Ketones rise as glucose and insulin levels fall. Low insulin allows the liver to make ketone bodies from fat stores to feed the brain. Ketones are like a specialized lipid jet fuel and are the main catalyst for synthesizing fatty acids in the infant's quickly growing brain. The heart also likes ketones as they are a metabolically clean fuel for this anaerobic organ. The heart can also burn fatty acids for fuel but it's more difficult for the brain because fatty acids cannot cross the blood-brain barrier fast enough to allow a person to remain conscious-they must be converted to ketones. During starvation ketones can provide 66 percent of the brain's energy supplies. Because the brain is an energy hog it seems clear human fat stores coevolved with brain function. It appears the gut also coevolved to create fat stores easily for a built-in brain support system.

The brain takes up ketones through a monocarboxylic acid transporter, which ramps up ketone transport when ketones are liberated from fat stores. Cold temperatures empty fat cells and liberate fatty acids, which are rapidly changed to ketones for the brain to use. Cold also increases the brain's metabolic capacity by limiting the waste products burned. Ketones do not draw on protein stores as glucose does, thus protecting the integrity of organs. This is an evolutionary survival mechanism for cold environments.

I believe this design goes all the way back to our mammalian ancestors who survived the K-T event on a diet filled with marine food and little else. This would have made them adapt to an environment that selected for cold and the Epi-paleo Rx. I think as time marched on from the K-T event, mammals readapted to longer light cycles and the presence of carbohydrates as the land recovered from the global catastrophe.

The only factor that limits the use of ketones by the brain is the rate of ketone production by the liver. This is why liver function is tightly linked to brain function. Liver disease in humans leads to hepatic encephalopathy, a worsening of brain function that occurs when the liver can no longer detoxify the blood. Once you think about how the gut and the brain coevolved you can make huge clinical strides in treating diseases. The road to optimal human health requires making sure these two organs function as designed.

Based on this coevolution, the basis of the Epi-paleo template requires seafood and fat to be a large part of the diet. This diet was formative to our species and we have gotten away from it for too long. The road back to your best starts where evolution sculpted the changes in gut and the brain that made us into modern humans.

Other environmental factors have also been found to influence the expression of our DNA, a phenomenon called epigenetics. Epigenetics is now thought to play a larger role than our genes do. How our genes are expressed has more to do with who we are then the original copy of genes we were born with.

Remember from the Hormone 101 blog post, we need sufficient vitamin A and T3 to convert LDL cholesterol to pregnenolone, a precursor to a chain of other hormones in the body. That chain ends in vitamin D. DHA, vitamin A, and vitamin D have long served as environmental signals to our brain. DHA and vitamin A have a 600-million-year history as cosensors in the visual system of all species. Vitamin A goes back 3 billion years to blue algae and was modified when photosynthesis first evolved. Vitamin D appears to go back 750 million years as the first natural sun screen. Over time we have not really increased the number of receptors but we have given them many more functions as biology has become more complex. This suggests these variables are very important for the regulation of the brain and the gut. Modern gastroenterology and neuroscience research is pointing us in this very direction, although modern medicine is not.

This makes reading the steroid pathways' response to inflammation the Rosetta stone for monitoring human health. We need to think of food as hormone information, not as a metabolic fuel. Think of the Epi-paleo Rx as human jet fuel for the nervous system because we go where the brain goes. Think of the gastrointestinal tract as a metabolic computer that adjusts your physiology in response to the nutrients it detects. This is how the brain-gut axis works in humans.

HOW TO CONSIDER EATING

The Epi-paleo Rx for optimal human health

- Always respect circadian cycles and eat according to season
- Lots of good quality proteins (see below)
- Lots of good quality fats (grass-fed/pastured animal fats, lard, tallow)
- Liberal uses of seafood broths and bone broth made from ocean and grass-fed animals (to heal the gut)
- Fermented vegetables and/or probiotics (to repopulate the gut for optimal human flora)

THE BASE OF THE PROTEIN/FAT PYRAMID OF THE EPI-PALEO RX

This diet is the best at controlling inflammation at the brain level to affect hormonal modulation and epigenetic expression.

The levels of the pyramid are ordered from best choice for the human brain to next best.

1. The base of the pyramid is shellfish (oysters) other than crustaceans. They are the most nutrient-dense of any food for optimal brain function.

2. Crustaceans

3. Fish

4. Offal, or organ meats, of pastured/grass-fed animals. This is where micronutrient density is greatest in meats but not seafood!

5. The fifth level of the pyramid is where modern-day Paleo begins: Grass-fed skeletal meats.

6. Pastured eggs if there are no contraindications of inflammation, such as autoimmunity.*

7. Seeds and nuts.* Leaning toward omega 3 nuts is fine but this becomes important if there is a serious EFA imbalance only on direct testing.

FATS: (IN ORDER OF OPTIMAL)

1. Spring and summer: Coconut oil, ghee, palm oil, duck fat, beef tallow, bacon fat, duck fat, pastured butter if there are no medical issue precluding its use, olive or avocado oils for salads, macadamia nut oils for mayonnaise, raw cream if there are no contraindications.* When you eat seafood try to use MUFAs as the added fat.

2. Fall and Winter: ghee, pastured butter, duck fat, beef tallow, bacon fat, non-hydrogenated lard, raw cream.* Stick to animal fats in colder months. When you eat seafood try to use MUFAs as the added fat.*

3. When you eat non-seafood protein you should add saturated fats to your diet to the greatest degree! Grass-fed red meat and offal come packed with saturated fats and fish do not, as I explained in the webinar. When I eat non-seafood protein and saturated fats I also add sea vegetables to the meal. The healthy human colon converts complex carbohydrates to short-chain fatty acids (SCFA) to increase omega 3 content in our colon and diminish the risk of diverticulitis and colon cancer. This is only done when gut microflora function well, however this process can be re engineered by evolutionary dietary modifications.

*These were covered in depth in the webinar on this topic for members of our community.

FOODS I TOTALLY ELIMINATE FROM THE EPI-PALEO RX:

1. All grains, no matter how they are prepared culturally.

2. All U.S. dairy (including raw dairy) because of the A1 casein problem, its ties to BCM-7 (a detrimental opiate), and its massive link to Hashimoto's and disease. One can use French or New Zealand dairy products.

3. All nightshades vegetables if you have chronic inflammation and low vitamin D: Datura, Mandragora (mandrake), Atropa belladonna (deadly nightshade), Lycium barbarum (wolfberry), Physalis philadelphica (tomatillo), Physalis peruviana (Cape gooseberry flower), Capsicum (chili pepper, bell pepper), Solanum (potato, tomato, eggplant), Nicotiana (tobacco), and Petunia. With the exception of tobacco (Nicotianoideae) and petunia (Petunioideae), most of the economically important genera are contained in the subfamily Solanaceae. READ MY CAVEAT BELOW ABOUT THE DIETARY USES!

Many members of the Solanaceae family are used by humans and are important sources of food, spice, and medicine. However, Solanaceae species are often rich in alkaloids with a toxicity to humans and animals that ranges from mildly irritating (most) to fatal in small quantities.

What are Solanaceae? If you have an autoimmunity, degenerative disc disease, or degenerative joint disease consider avoiding them:

A. American-grown soy! It has been hybridized with petunias, a nightshade, to be pesticide resistant (Round-Up)

B. All potatoes (NOTE: this does not include sweet potatoes because they are from the Marigold family)

C. Tomatoes (green are worse than any other type. Eating other red fruits of veggies offsets the lycopene issue. Watermelon, for example, blows tomatoes away as a source of lycopene.)

D. Eggplant

E. Sweet and hot peppers (including paprika, cayenne pepper, and Tabasco sauce, but not black pepper)

F. Ground cherries

G. Tomatillos and tamarillos

H. Garden huckleberry and naranjillas

I. Pepinos and pimentos

J. Only the cape gooseberry is a nightshade (Physalis peruviana). Most gooseberries are not in the nightshade family. They are in the genus Ribes and are related to currants.

K. Blueberries, strawberries, okra, and artichokes, have some solanaceae toxin in them, but are not strict nightshades. If you have arthritis or another inflammatory condition you might want to rethink the dogma that surrounds them (kills me to tell you this).

CAVEAT

The key point to consider and why I use some of these veggies and fruits in my Epi-paleo Rx e-cookbook: Most of the foods listed above have small amounts of the toxins in them. If you are ill with debilitating arthritis, Hashimoto's or any autoimmune disease, fibromyalgia, biotoxin illness, or just have a high HS CRP, seriously consider limiting these foods. In many countries around the world people have found a way around these toxins by slow cooking their nightshades at very low temperatures for long periods of time. This keeps the vitamins intact while making the fruits easier on the body. I use nightshades in my sauces in this way. Nightshades have oxalic acid, which depletes the calcium in your body. Dairy has a lot of calcium, and if tomatoes take it away from our body, why not consider having them together to create a balanced dietary effect? This is why many Italian dishes are prepared with a combination of the two. As most of you know, I am no fan of A1 dairy products for many reasons I laid out in the Epi-paleo Webinar (such as BCM-7 casein and DPP-IV), but if you learn how to create a balanced environment in your body then you don't need to avoid the foods you love. This is what

I learned by doing quarterly testing on myself more than seven years. When I saw my HS CRP and Vitamin D were unaffected by some of these things I ate them without regret and you should, too. That being said, if you have an inflammatory condition, like most patients in my clinic do, you need to rethink this food group carefully.

Most of my spine patients with degenerative disc or joint disease are shocked by this information. Most have never heard it before.

4. All fruits when they are out of season for your particular geography. When in season they are fine for you.

5. Optional: Cut out all poultry and fowl. For optimal health limit fowl if you can afford to. All fowl should be eliminated until you're healthy, with the exception of duck. Personally, I eat very little fowl but when I do it is wild duck, quail, or pheasant. I use more duck fat than meat.

6. All legumes without exception, even for cultural reasons.

7. Any foods containing saponin . Alfalfa sprouts, yucca, soy, quilla extract (used to foam drinks like beer), and chia seeds.

8. Avoid all sweeteners, period. Stevia is OK (I rarely use it now) if it has no maltodextrin or other additives.

9. When eating non-ocean fats or protein consider adding sea veggies to the recipe (www.theseaweedman.com is a good online source of seaweeds).

A. Irish Moss (Chondrus crispus, carrageen) is full of electrolyte minerals, such as calcium, magnesium, sodium and potassium. Its mucilaginous compounds help detoxification, boost metabolism, and strengthen hair, skin and nails. In Eastern medicine it is traditionally used for a low sex drive because it helps support T3 levels to convert LDL to progesterone and not to cortisol.

B. Wakame (Alaria, Undaria) is a high-protein, high-calcium seaweed, with carotenes, iron, and vitamin C. It is used in Chinese medicine for hair growth and luster and for skin tone because it optimizes thyroid function.

C. Kelp (Laminaria) contains the fat-soluble vitamins A, B, E, D and K in high quantity, and is a major source of vitamin C from the sea. It also happens to be rich in many minerals found in land-based plants. This is why it made my top-10 supplement list long ago in the blog series. Kelp proteins are high quality and present in abundance for a sea plant. Kelp contains sodium alginate (algin), an element that helps remove radioactive particles (think Fukishima iodine) and heavy metals from the body. Kelp can work as a blood purifier, relieve arthritis stiffness, and promotes adrenal, pituitary, and thyroid health. Kelp's natural iodine can normalize thyroid-related disorders such as obesity and muscle fatigue seen in fibromyalgia cases. Clinical pearl for people with herpes virus of any type: It is a demulcent that helps eliminate herpes outbreaks after they have occurred. Kelp is nutrient-rich and a small amount often gives large clinical results.

D. Hijiki is a mineral-rich, high-fiber seaweed that contains 20 percent protein, vitamin A, carotenes and calcium. Hijiki has the most calcium of any sea green-1400 mg per 100 grams of dry weight.

E. Kombu (laminaria digitata, setchelli, horsetail kelp) has a long tradition as a Japanese delicacy with nutritional healing value. Natural healers use it is a decongestant for excess mucous and to help normalize blood pressure. It has abundant iodine, carotenes, B, C, D and E vitamins, minerals like calcium, magnesium, potassium, silica, iron and zinc, and the powerful skin healing nutrient germanium, which is a rare element in the human diet. Kombu is a meaty, high-protein seaweed. It is higher in natural mineral salts than most other seaweeds. I often add a strip of kombu to my bone broths and seafood broths.

F. Nori (porphyra, laver) is a red sea plant with a sweet, meaty taste when dried. It contains nearly 50 percent balanced protein that is easy to assimilate, higher than any other sea plant. Nori's fiber makes it popular for sushi wrapping. I do not eat any rice because its microRNA directly affect our DNA expression. Nori is rich in all the carotenes, calcium, iodine, iron, and phosphorus.

G. Sea palm (Postelsia palmaeformis), or American arame, grows only on the Pacific Coast of North America by Oregon and Washington State. It has a honeyed, salty taste that makes it a tasty vegetable. I like it with my cauliflower rice recipe from the e-cookbook, or as a summer or autumn salad topping.

H. Bladderwrack is loaded with vitamin K and it is an excellent adrenal adaptogen. It helps sensitize us to insulin because of its K2-like effects. It is often used today by Native American cultures in broths and in sauna and steam baths for degenerative arthritis and inflammatory joint conditions.

I. Dulse (Palmaria palmata), a red sea plant, is very rich in iron. The last two sea veggies are my favorites because they have the most iodine of any plants on our planet. It also has abundant protein and vitamin A. What really makes it a good balanced nutrient for a lactovegetarian Paleo diet is that it contains 300 times more iodine and 50 times more iron than wheat products. Tests on dulse show antiviral action against the herpes virus.

J. Arame (Eisenia bycyclis), is one of the ocean's richest sources of iodine. It often contains more iodine than seafood does! Because of its high iodine content it can have major effects on a woman's progesterone to estradiol ratio. If you are estrogen dominant you might consider using this as a staple in your broths and recipes. Many natural healers use arame to help reduce breast and uterine fibroids, excessive bleeding, fibrocystic disease of the breasts, and ovarian cysts. It is also quite helpful in cases of PCOS with acne and excessive facial hair. It contains fat-soluble vitamins and phytohormones, which can help normalize perimenopausal and menopausal symptoms. Arame is often associated with soft, wrinkle-free skin, enhanced hair growth, and an incredible sheen to hair. This sea veggie increases your free T3 to a dramatic degree when used regularly in your diet.

I focus on those who are not well or as ideal as they want to be. Those of you who heard the July 2012 webinar got quite a bit more data behind these simple recommendations. Share them with your loved ones and then post your results at my blog as time evolves. Your comments are important to people who come read it in the future.

Also, smile at someone. A smile is the lighting system of the face, the cooling system of the head, and the heating system of the heart. This will help lower your cortisol too and help you get well. This is part of the Epi-paleo Rx as well.

There's a huge difference between the Paleo diet and Epi-paleo Rx when you are not well. The Paleo template is a very good diet because it is better at controlling inflammation than most other diets. However, I discovered the Epi-paleo Rx seven years ago as I kept researching the biochemistry of diet in those with serious diseases and inflammation. It destroys inflammation while providing massive quantities of brain-specific nutrients to rebuild your neural circuitry. The Epi-paleo Rx is based on how we evolved from transitional apes. You decide now what you want to be with your diet: effective or correct.

I'm just the guy with the flashlight on the road to optimal.

J. Arame seawead

theseaweedman.com

Irish sea moss

Wakame

Kelp

Kombu

Nori

Appendix B

THE COLD THERAPY RX

WHAT IS THE NEXT STEP IN THE EVOLUTION OF THE EPI-PALEO RX?

The cold thermogenesis protocol should added gradually to the Epi-paleo Rx protocol. I hope you all realize that not everyone will need it. Some will need it because they have special needs, including gastric bypass patients, HCG users, those on exogenous steroids, chronic pain patients, and those with metabolic syndrome type 2 diabetes as a few examples.

Prolonged and controlled local peripheral skin cooling can induce selective "damage" and increased hypothalamic signaling by forcing adipocyte apoptosis and subsequent loss of subcutaneous fat, without damaging the overlying skin or the underlying muscle layers. This means acute cold causes rapid leptin sensitivity! It means fat is forced to liberate leptin from fat cells to slowly lower its serum levels as long as the cold stimulus is applied safely. This is new scientific information that was first carried out in pigs in 2008 and subsequently tested in humans and found to be quite effective for fat removal in certain selected areas of the body. Maintenance of a normal temperature and the normal variations of the circadian and lunar rhythms are achieved by changes in all physiological systems, one of the most important of which is alteration in skin blood flow in humans. My version of cold thermogenesis for the Epi-paleo Rx generalizes these effects for the entire body to force the brain to slowly rewire in the hypothalamus to burn all excessive white adipose tissue (WAT) by inducing the formation of brown adipose tissue (BAT) using cold alone.

A cursory version was first popularized by Ray Cronise in 2010 and by Tim Ferriss in 2011 but neither one of them took this process to its biological end point for permanent fat loss. I have done an epic 18 month bio-hack on this very topic. I believe what I have found has profound and wide clinical applications for us all.

Moreover, neither of these men realized the dietary forces that can be used with cold therapy to produce dramatic results. Cold is not just a fat loss tool. It has several other benefits to human physiology. I believe the reason for this is because the hypothalamic biology is not well appreciated by most scientists today. When you sustain this process, steepen and expand the temperature gradient across a larger surface area, and specifically alter the macronutrient ratios, some amazing things become possible. I share with you how cold thermogenesis can augment the Epi-paleo Rx reset and can make a huge difference to those with vagal nerve damage who do not get a large bang from my standard reset.

If you have a gastric bypass, type 2 diabetes, chronic pain, adrenal fatigue, or poor sleep cold therapy will likely shock you at how well it helps you. NASA data from the 1970s has shown that fasted mammals cannot increase glucose turnover rate when cold adapted. They also cannot increase their muscle glucose uptake when exposed to cold environments because the cold enhances the supply of fatty acids and ketone bodies to muscles during exercise. I have tested this on myself for the last 18 months to look for all the pitfalls I could muster. Before you begin you must make sure your cardiac risks are low and talk things over with your doctor and family. Most people will have no trouble doing this at home.

LET US LEARN THE BEST WAY TO COLD ADAPT FOR THE EPI-PALEO RX RESET NOW

When I began this I did a lot or reading on training of NASA astronaut, Special Ops and Navy Seal. You first must choose what environment to which you want to cold adapt. Cold water immersion dictates a more rapid drop in surface and core temperature than exposure to cold air. So most people will choose to use water because it works a lot faster. Before you start, always eat a high-fat (MCT>saturated fats>MUFAs>PUFAs) and/or protein meal right before you attempt to cold adapt. Also, drink 16-32 ounces of ice cold water immediately prior to the test no matter what stage you are at. Why? Your body temperature is incredibly hot at approximately 98.6 degrees Fahrenheit, and ice water is approximately 40 degrees Fahrenheit. In order to maintain this homeostasis, your body has to bring that ice water up by about 60 degrees, and, by definition, it takes 1 calorie to raise the temperature of 1 liter of water by approximately 2 degrees. That means to raise the temperature of 1 liter of ice water by 60 degrees Fahrenheit, your body would burn about 30 calories. Two liters, which is about eight glasses of water, would burn 60 calories. Do not drink more than 32 oucnes of water before this test because cold adaptation also affects our thirst centers. You should always consider drinking cold liquids as part of your dietary plan as it can increase your metabolic rate by 30-40%. If you get a lot of brain freezes when you drink cold things this might signal you suffer from a high tissue omega six level. You need to proceed with caution while trying to apply cold thermogenesis. You will see why your omega 6 level matters soon.

I usually will do my training in the morning at sunrise or at night after dinner. I do not recommend trying this on an empty stomach. In the beginning of my adaptation I also used bitter melon extract to cold adapt. Bitter melon appears to be quite effective at creating BAT from WAT, especially in those with type 2 diabetes or metabolic syndrome. No one knows why it really works but I believe it is has to do with the loss of adiponectin and leptin from fat cells with the simultaneous induction of Irisin from the cold stimulus on the skin and subcutaneous fat.

Step 1

Cold adaptation occurs 100 times faster using metal over air. But this is far too dangerous to use at home, so never try it. Water is 24 times more effective than just cold air. You need a simple skin thermometer, ice, a bathroom sink and a watch with a timer. How does one cool the skin but not the core? Simply monitor your skin temperature as it goes from its normal temperature in your house until it gets to 50-55 degrees Fahrenheit while in your cold environment on your skin surface and maintain it there. Go no lower. When you get there, watch your skin color when it begins to get to pink or white as its going south of 50-55 degrees. End the session then. In the beginning your sessions will end faster than later because you're cold adapting.

The easiest way to cold adapt is to first place just your face first in ice cold water. You must not use any makeup or facial products. Just submerge your face into water in a sink or bowl of water with ice. Wait until the water is between 50-55 degrees and enter face first and see how long you can tolerate it using a time piece. Record the time. For the next two weeks work your way up increasing the time your face is submerged until you need to take a breath. The rate of adaptation to this will vary for people. When you finish this proceed to number two.

Step 2

Buy a compression shirt that is quite tight and begin to place 20 or 40 pounds of ice on your torso. Double bag the ice to stop leakage on clothing or furniture. Compression shirts collapses the surface capillaries and allows your skin temps to fall faster, quickly sensitizing you to cold. Initially this will be tough but you will adapt to it in time. Try to extend your time 5 minutes each session until you get to 60 minutes. You will notice your skin is pink to cherry read and numb in places. When you get to 60 minutes then take the compression shirt off for further testing. Place the direct plastic ice bags on your skin now and repeat the skin cooling. If you develop cold urticaria (hives or welts) at this time, this is a sign you have high levels of tissue and serum omega-6 content. Stop the experiment and follow a ketogenic Paleolithic diet until you have a blood omega 6 to 3 ratio that is below 10 to 1. You can also test your serum for this ratio. If you do not develop cold urticaria proceed on to see how long you can tolerate the cold. Make sure you have no metal on your torso, ears or nose when you do this. Record your times. Pay attention to your skin color. After 10 minutes you will notice numbness and tingling on these cold areas. As you increase your times increase you may notice numbness in areas adjacent to the iced areas. This usually occurs with longer exposures and with more surface area covered. The length of time you expose yourself should be matched to your BMI. The fatter you are the longer your exposure should be. You want your skin to always remain pink to cherry red when you are doing this. If it gets white you need to stop the test and take a warm shower. Do these things indoors initially where you can control the air temperature during adaptation. Do not start this outside until you cold adapt for at least a month. When you can tolerate the skin being covered for one hour with pink to cherry red skin you're now ready for the Cold Tub step.

Step 3

Once you complete Step 2, you can try cold showers to ready your body for immersion, but I did not use this much when I was training my brain to rewire. I went straight to the bathtub and filled it with cold tap water. With immersion, the major heat exchange in water occurs by means of conduction with the surrounding water. The exceptions to this are the non-immersed body parts, in most cases the head. The head can represent a significant site of heat loss to the environment owing to its minimal insulation (small fat layers) and lack of vasoconstriction in the scalp.

I then add 20 pounds of ice to my chest and abdomen region while my body is in the tub. Initially I kept my socks and gloves on my extremities and I wore a knitted cap. This was to combat the vasoconstriction that normally occurs in the extremities. The hat was to keep in heat from the veins of the scalp to allow for an adaptation to immersion. This step will take you some time to get used too. You lose 20-40 percent more heat from cerebral blood shunting when you cool adapt. After I was adapted to 20 pounds of ice (about 5-7 days) then I removed socks, gloves and head cap. If you get lightheaded this means you're not ready for the tub. Abort the tub and go back to dunking your face in the cold water. If you can handle the 20 pounds of ice you can increase it 10 pounds of ice at a time to cover more of your body with icy water. If you have access to skin thermometers (I did) that an anesthesiologist would normally use during a surgery, you are looking to get your skin surface temp to 50-55 degrees. A patient told me we can buy them online. We are trying to use the peripheral nervous system's cold receptors in the skin to tell the brain something has radically changed in our current environment. After you can get past 45 minutes of this you will notice your tolerance to cold dramatically changes in water, air, and in ice. You will be able to wear less clothing and go outside and not be cold. In fact you may notice your temperature rises in anticipation of the cold tub. I do this now all the time. You will be able to drive on the highway with the windows down in the dead of the winter and feel amazing. Your significant other will notice you seem to radiate heat at rest when you lay down to sleep. The longer you tolerate this situation, the better adaptations you will get. The extent of the training depends upon your goal.

Step 4

At 45 minutes you can choose to stop and then plan on doing this 2-5 times a week depending upon your starting weight, body fat percent, and goals. You also need to be cognizant of where you want to lose the fat on your body. If you have it in your belly, butt, and legs continue using the indoor tub or an outdoor lake or pool. Immersion is the best way to shed body fat and regain leptin sensitivity. Once you can accomplish this in your house for one month you can than move to the outdoors if you like. If you have a pool, lake or hot tub you can set its temp lower to replace the ice use. I tend to use the lake or my hot tub, but I use them differently. When I want a quick training to maintain my adaptation I just jump into the lake for a 10-20 minutes from my neck down. I pay attention to my skin color as I do this. The hardest part is emerging from the lake and walking back to the house and not being in the water. It is easier now for me but in the beginning it was tough. Most of the time I use my hot tub to train. I get in it and I cold adapt my upper body with ice bags on my torso while my bottom half is submerged in the water. I alter the water temps to higher than my torso because I have very little fat on this part of lower parts of my body today. So often I will sit in warmer water while my upper half is completely exposed to the elements with ice on my chest and abdomen. It is very effective at lowering your surface temperatures to 50-55 degrees in 2-3 minutes. This augments thermogenesis naturally using convection currents of different temperatures. I can do this for amazing lengths of time now after 18 months of training.

Do not try to bite off more than you can chew. Heat spontaneously tends to flows from a body at a higher temperature to a body at a lower temperature. So a warmer lower body and a 50 degree skin temp on the torso create a dynamic that makes using cold thermogenesis really easy daily. Anyone who as soaked in a volcanic geothermal spring can tell you they hardly notice the cold on their exposed. This method is really effective at increasing thermogenesis in the exposed areas for fat loss. If you have a lot of belly fat this is not your best method, but it will still work. If you have torso, back, facial, neck fat (sleep apnea) this works like a charm quickly.

Step 5

You burn a lot more calories when it's cold outside so you MUST get outside in cold and try not to wear a ton of clothing as you adapt. In the beginning, most wear a ton of clothing when they go outside in cold weather. That slows adaptation to cold. According to Andrew J. Young, Ph.D., of the U.S. Army Research Institute of Environmental Medicine in Natick, Mass., "There are two factors that could cause energy expenditure to increase with falling outdoor temperature. First, if shivering is elicited by cold, then energy expenditure increases. However, different people have differing shivering-response sensitivity, and intensity of shivering will be influenced by magnitude of decrease in body (deep core and skin) temperature, which in turn is influenced by body size and fat content that vary widely among people, as well as clothing worn. So some folks don't shiver at all (too warmly dressed, excessive body fat, leptin resistance), and a man in the cold is not always a cold man. The more leptin resistance one is the more you should consider a steeper slope of adaptation to lose fat.

The other reason energy expenditure might increase in cold weather is if you perform heavy physical labor like weight lifting or walking in deep snow. Additionally, there is a likelihood that you could have a slight increase in calorie burn (about 3 to 7 percent) from your body re-warming itself from cold air touching your skin and warming the cold air that goes into your lungs. This is also why when I emerge from my cold tub, lake or ice baths I will remain outside in the buff for several minutes to really heighten the cold stimulus. I immediately go inside to a warm terrycloth robe, which captures my thermal loss and increases caloric burn for about an hour after the cooling. This is a great time to work out as well. You will also notice your ability to lift and workout increases by 5-10 percent. Recovery is simply stunning. You won't believe what a cold tub does after a serious high intensity work out. Your recovery will amaze you and you sleep will be shockingly solid. Nothing is better to induce sleep in my view than cold thermogenesis induction.

The beauty of this adaptation is that is does not require any change to your core temps. When you begin to mess with your core temps you can get into trouble with frostbite and freezing injury. The higher your omega-6 content the worse cold adapted you will be. The higher your omega-3 content the better you will adapt to cold. The higher protein/fat intake you have the slower you will adapt to cold. The more carbs your have in your diet (leptin resistance) the easier you will find it to adapt to cold. If you have a history of smoking, dipping, cigar use you will not cold adapt well. If you are dehydrated (booze/wine) you will not cold adapt fast either.

Step 6

If you use just air to adapt to cold thermogenesis it will take a lot longer but there is one thing I should mention. Slowly remove clothing as you proceed over time. As you remove clothing there is a specific way you should pick the clothes to remove. You want to expose your face and head to cold as soon as possible. Remember, when in number one we begin cold water adaptation to our face. This is because all mammals have a reflex called a dive reflex that is built in because we all were formed in a fluid filled placenta. When we expose ourselves to cold on our face first we stimulate slowing of our heart rate. This is soon followed by vasoconstriction of blood flow in our extremities. When we continue to dive deep we force blood and water to pass through our organs and endothelium to fill our air filled cavities like our chest. This has been experimentally shown in humans during deep water cold dives. We actually drown in pulmonary fluids but can still survive! As a physician, I see this problem daily in our ICUs in patients with ARDS. Sadly, we do not treat them as I think we should given what we know about the mammalian dive reflex, but that is another story. Do not worry I do not plan to use this adaptation in my reset in the near future! I'd love to try it but I hear it takes years to perfect.

When you first begin cold training with clothing on, the way you disrobe when you re-enter a warm environment also matters for the adaptation to become more comfortable and less agonizing. So first expose your face, then your head to the warm environment. Then expose your extremities to re establish the blood flow and lastly your torso and abdomen. This progression of re-exposure to the warm environment from the cold will make it more bearable as time progresses. If you remove clothing in a different layered fashion you can abruptly increase cortisol release to cause a vascular instability. This instability is felt to be behind a thermal dump that underpins vascular reperfusion injuries seen in frostbite and hypothermia injuries. If you are not overheated by heavy clothing or your warming environment, the cold (when other symptoms are warm) will trigger non-shivering thermogenesis to be induced and you will continue to burn calories as free heat for many hours after the cold exposure. This is why people who are in cold environments tend to be quite thin when they are eating a non-Western diet. You will also notice a change in your hunger and appetite, because they will decline. This addition is also quite beneficial to those with binge eating disorders too.

I believe that cold thermogenesis is an evolutionary forerunner for all mammalian physiology before exercise was evolved or naturally selected for in mammals. This is a controversial point but I think based upon what we know to be true today it's not a fringe theory. The available food sources also helped simultaneously sculpt evolutionary pressures that were naturally selected for in a cold environment. I believe natural exercise was selected for by movements to warmer environments, longer light cycles, and more abundant carbohydrates in the environment. Mammals did not first evolve predominately in warm environments. Humans certainly might have evolved this way...but we are descended from these eutherian mammals and their epigenetic programs remain buried within us but are just not selected for these days. When we induce the programs, what this may mean for us today is among the most exciting things in biology I have come across in 30 years. It appears cold thermogenesis not only opens a novel metabolic pathway in modern mammals and humans but it also activates our longevity genes. Many of the things aging researchers and scientist currently hold to as core beliefs may in fact not be true. The ability to test these theories is now here because of how we are unfolding the story of our own biology using a piece-by-piece approach that the QUILT provides.

Consider this: A 26.2 mile marathon burns 2,600 calories. My three-hour training session I did this morning burned 3,800 calories. The cold effect on weight loss is great, but what excites me more is which form of exercise do you think might cause more harm in the long run? One thought might just alter your DNA!

REFERENCES

1. Selective cryolysis: A novel method of non-invasive fat removal (pages 595–604) Dieter Manstein, Hans Laubach, Kanna Watanabe, William Farinelli, David Zurakowski and R. Rox Anderson Article first published online: 24 OCT 2008 | DOI: 10.1002/lsm.20719
2. http://abcnews.go.com/Health/story?id=4393377&page=1#.TzX9JJjMpN1
3. Hassi, J.; Mäkinen, T.M.; Rintamäki, H. (2005) Prediction and Prevention of Frostbite. In Prevention of Cold Injuries (pp. KN1-1 – KN1-10). Meeting Proceedings RTO-MP-HFM-126, Keynote 1. Neuilly-sur-Seine, France: RTO. Available from: http://www.rto.nato.int/abstracts.asp.
4. Boström PA, et al., "PGC1-a-dependent myokine that drives brown-fat-like development of white fat and thermogenesis," Nature. 2012 Jan 11. doi: 10.1038/nature10777.
5. http://www.nejm.org/doi/full/10.1056/NEJMoa0808718

6. http://www.nap.edu/openbook.php?record_id=5197&page=127

7. Liu et al.: "Fasting Activation of AgRP Neurons Requires NMDA Receptors and Involves Spinogenesis and Increased Excitatory Tone." Neuron, DOI:10.1016/j.neuron.2011.11.027

8. http://abcnews.go.com/Health/Wellness/nasa-scientist-chills-body-shed-pounds/story?id=12000983#.TzXxpJjMq8V

9. Tong Shi, et al. "SIRT3, a Mitochondrial Sirtuin Deacetylase, Regulates Mitochondrial Function and Thermogenesis in Brown Adipocytes," J. Biol. Chem., Vol. 280, No. 14, Issue of April 8, pp. 13560–13567, 2005

10. http://abcnews.go.com/Health/freezing-fat-fda-green-lights-weight-loss-treatment/story?id=11641994#.TzXx2ZjMq8U

Made in United States
North Haven, CT
02 June 2023